MINIMUM SYSTEM REQUIREMENTS

Windows

233 MHz processor
128 MB of RAM (256 MB of RAM recommended)
800 x 600 resolution monitor
Windows 2000/XP/Vista
8x CD-ROM drive
20 MB of available hard disk space

LICENSE AGREEMENT

1. F.A. Davis ("FAD") grants the purchaser of *MA Review Notes: Exam Certification Pocket Guide* limited license for the program on the enclosed CD-ROM ("Software"). FAD retains complete copyright to the Software and associated content.
2. Licensee has nonexclusive right to use this copy of the Software on one device on one screen at one location. Any other use is forbidden.
3. Licensee may physically transfer the Software from one computer to another, provided that it is used on only one computer at any one time. Except for the initial loading of the Software on a hard disk or for archival or backup purposes, Licensee may not copy, electronically transfer, or otherwise distribute copies.
4. This License Agreement automatically terminates if Licensee fails to comply with any term of this Agreement.
5. SOFTWARE UPDATES. Updated versions of the Software may be created or issued by FAD from time to time. At its sole option, FAD may make such updates available to the Licensee or authorized transferees who have returned the registration card, paid the update fee, and returned the original CD-ROM to FAD.

Limited Warranty and Disclaimer

ırnished will be
very to you by
receipt shall be
ıanying materi-
ꞔ complete risk
is with you.

FAD makes no warranty that the Software will meet your requirements or that Software operation will be uninterrupted or error free or that Software defects are correctable. No oral or written information or advice given by FAD, its dealers, distributors, agents, or employees shall create warranty or in any way increase the scope of this limited warranty.

REMEDIES. FAD's entire liability and your exclusive remedy shall be limited to replacing the defective media if returned to FAD (at your expense) accompanied by dated proof of purchase satisfactory to FAD not later than one week after the end of the warranty period, provided you have first received a Return Authorization by calling or writing FAD in advance. The maximum liability of FAD and its licensors shall be the purchase price of the software. In no event shall FAD and its licensors be liable to you or any other person for any direct, indirect, incidental, consequential, special, exemplary, or punitive damages for tort, contract, strict liability, or other theory arising out of the use of, or inability to use the software.

ENTIRE AGREEMENT. This Agreement contains the entire understanding of the parties hereto relating to the subject matter hereof and supersedes all prior representations or agreements.

GOVERNING LAW. This Agreement and Limited Warranty are governed by the laws of the Commonwealth of Pennsylvania. All warranty matters should be addressed to:
F.A. Davis, Publishers, 1915 Arch Street, Philadelphia, PA 19103

INSTALLATION INSTRUCTIONS

Windows

Step 1. Insert CD into your CD-ROM drive.
Step 2. After a few moments, the CD-ROM menu will automatically open.
Step 3. Select the item to install.

If the CD-ROM Menu does not automatically open, from the START Menu, select RUN and enter X:\setup.exe (where "X" is the letter of your CD-ROM drive) and select OK

For Technical Support, e-mail: support@fadavis.com

MA Review Notes

Exam Certification Pocket Guide

Susan Perreira, MS, CMA, RMA

Purchase additional copies of this book at your health science bookstore or directly from F.A. Davis by shopping online at www.fadavis.com or by calling 800-323-3555 (US) or 800-665-1148 (CAN)

A Davis's Notes Book

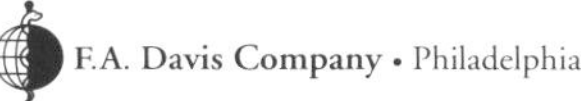

F. A. Davis Company
1915 Arch Street
Philadelphia, PA 19103
www.fadavis.com

Printed in China

Last digit indicates print number: 10 9 8 7 6 5 4 3 2 1

Acquisitions Editor: Andy McPhee
Manager of Content Development: George Lang
Senior Developmental Editor: Jennifer Pine
Art and Design Manager: Carolyn O'Brien

Reviewers: Tricia Berry, MATL, BSOT, OTR/L; Carole Berube, MA, MSN, BSN, RN; Carmen Carpenter, CMA, RN, MS; Renea Craven, MLT, RMA, CLS; Robyn Gohsman, AAS, RMA, CMAS; Sue A. Hunt, MA, RN, CMA; Deborah S. Janeczko, MA-CTE, RMA; Betty J. Klein, MS, RN; Joyce A. Minton, MA Education, CMA, RMA; Evierlee O'Nan, RMA, EMT-B; Carol D. Tamparo, CMA-A, PhD; Deborah L. White, AS, CMA, BHS, MS/HPE

Look for our other Davis's Notes Titles

Coding Notes: Medical Insurance Pocket Guide
ISBN-10: 0-8036-1536-1 / ISBN-13: 978-0-8036-1536-6

Derm Notes: Dermatology Clinical Pocket Guide
ISBN-10: 0-8036-1495-0 / ISBN-13: 978-0-8036-1495-6

ECG Notes: Interpretation and Management Guide
ISBN-10: 0-8036-1347-4 / ISBN-13: 978-0-8036-1347-8

LabNotes: Guide to Lab and Diagnostic Tests
ISBN-10: 0-8036-1265-6 / ISBN-13: 978-0-8036-1265-5

NutriNotes: Nutrition & Diet Therapy Pocket Guide
ISBN-10: 0-8036-1114-5 / ISBN-13: 978-0-8036-1114-6

MA Notes: Medical Assistant's Pocket Guide
ISBN-10: 0-8036-1281-8 / ISBN-13: 978-0-8036-1281-5

Ortho Notes: Clinical Examination Pocket Guide
ISBN-10: 0-8036-1350-4 / ISBN-13: 978-0-8036-1350-8

Provider's Coding Notes: Billing & Coding Pocket Guide
ISBN-10: 0-8036-1745-3 / ISBN-13: 978-0-8036-1745-2

PsychNotes: Clinical Pocket Guide
ISBN-10: 0-8036-1286-9 / ISBN-13: 978-0-8036-1286-0

Rehab Notes: Evaluation and Intervention Pocket Guide
ISBN-10: 0-8036-1398-9 /ISBN-13: 978-0-8036-1398-0

Respiratory Notes: Respiratory Therapist's Guide
ISBN-10: 0-8036-1467-5 / ISBN-13: 978-0-8036-1467-3

Screening Notes: Rehabilitation Specialists Pocket Guide
ISBN-10: 0-8036-1573-6 /ISBN-13: 978-0-8036-1573-1

Sport Notes: Rehabilitation Specialists Pocket Guide
ISBN-10: 0-8036-1875-1 /ISBN-13: 978-0-8036-1875-6

For a complete list of Davis's Notes and other titles for health care providers, visit www.fadavis.com.

Contacts • Phone/E-Mail

Name
Ph: e-mail:

Name
Ph: e-mail:

Name
Ph: e-mail:

Name
Ph: e-mail:

Name
Ph: e-mail:

Name
Ph: e-mail:

Name
Ph: e-mail:

Name
Ph: e-mail:

Name
Ph: e-mail:

Name
Ph: e-mail:

Name
Ph: e-mail:

Name
Ph: e-mail:

About the Author

The author received a Bachelor of Science degree in Education from Southern Connecticut State University in New Haven and a Master of Science degree in Allied Health from the University of Connecticut in Storrs. She is a Certified Medical Assistant through the American Association of Medical Assistants (AAMA) as well as a Registered Medical Assistant through the American Medical Technologists (AMT). In addition to over 9 years of experience in the field, she has been an educator for more than 25 years and currently serves as Professor and Department Coordinator for the Medical Assisting (MA) program at Capital Community College in Hartford, Connecticut. As an MA faculty member and field-experienced administrative and clinical MA, she recognizes fully the knowledge that newly graduated and experienced MAs must possess to become properly credentialed or recredentialed. As a result of her guidance, almost all graduates of her program pass either the CMA or RMA examination the first time, and she hopes that, with the help of *MA Review Notes,* the reader will pass the examination the first time too.

Benefits of Credentialing

- Attainment of a Certified Medical Assistant (CMA), Registered Medical Assistant (RMA), or Certified Medical Administrative Specialist (CMAS) credential confirms your in-depth knowledge of medical assisting and demonstrates your dedication to the field.
- Networking with other certified medical assistants, while earning Continuing Education Units (CEUs), may be cultivated by attending national conventions, state conventions, and local chapter meetings.
- The yearly income for a certified medical assistant (CMA, RMA, or CMAS) is higher than the employee wages of uncertified medical assistants.
- With national certification, there is no need to apply for reciprocity if you move out of state and wish to continue working in the field.
- Certification may not be mandated by law; however, more large medical facilities and outpatient offices are requiring medical assistants to be certified before possible employment.

- Today's medical employers recognize the value of and therefore seek certified medical assistants for the following reasons:
  1. Employee professionalism.
  2. Lower liability risk in several areas of their practices.
  3. Continuing complexity in the practice of medicine.
  4. Valuable ongoing contributions to the clinical and administrative ends of a given practice through continued education and recertification.

Book Features

This is a study guide containing all required areas of knowledge and will focus on essential key areas.

- It is written in an outline format.
- The candidate may add study notes to personalize their study guide.
- It's small enough in size to fit conveniently in a pocket or purse; candidates can refer to it whenever they have time throughout the day.
- It comes with an enclosed CD to give candidates an opportunity to test their knowledge at the end of any given tabbed section, and also includes simulated CMA, RMA, and CMAS examinations to take when they have completed their review study. These examinations will be timed and scored, with correct answers and rationales given when errors have been made.
- A candidate may retest at any time, as well as make changes to their notes. Overall, this will make study and test preparation easier and more productive.

Tips

Test Preparation

- The more prepared you are for the exam, the more confident you will be.
- Set up a study schedule for yourself and stick to it. Commit, commit, commit! Use 1.5 to 2 hours per day for consecutive days for a particular subject area (office, laboratory, clinical, anatomy, pharmacology, etc.).
- Organize your study time for each subject area.

1. Review competency skills.
2. Take notes (especially on information you have forgotten); create an outline format to your note-taking organizing your thoughts.
3. Note-taking will assist you in practicing memorization.

- Once you have studied an area (pharmacology, law and ethics, etc.), study the same information again to help reinforce your learning. Be OVERPREPARED!
- Drive and time the trip to the testing center a few days in advance to remove any anxiety about the center's location and the time it will take to get there. Plan to arrive early the day of the examination; you'll avoid being late due to traffic jams, etc.
- The night before the examination gather all the items you will need to bring with you to the examination (required identification[s], erasers, pencils, hard candy, etc.).
- The credentialing examinations are presented in a multiple-choice format, and you must choose an answer among four or five lettered response options. Incorrect response options are called *distractors*

1. Read each question and remember not to make assumptions by reading into the information presented. In other words, base your answer on the information provided.
2. Answer the question in your head before looking at the given response options.
3. Read the question a second time for full comprehension and then view the response options.
4. Remember, your initial response is usually the correct one, unless you did not fully comprehend the question.
5. If two or three response options are correct, check to see if the last given option is an "all the above" or a combination of previous options.
6. Usually, after ruling out some options you will be left with two possible answers; select the most correct one.
7. Pay special attention to questions containing words that have been **bolded**, *italicized,* <u>underlined</u>, or CAPITALIZED.
8. Watch out for words such as except, unless, unacceptable, avoid, contraindicated, or never that are used in a test question. These questions have a negative polarity, look for the one "negative" or "false" answer.

The following is an example of this type of question:

The five Cs of communication components are all the following ***except:***

A. consistent
B. clear
C. cohesive
D. concise
E. complete

In this case you need to identify which responses are components of communication in order to find the one response that is not. The response that is not a component is the correct answer.

9. Remember that this is a timed examination so you should have to spend less than a minute on each question. If the question asked lacks clarity for you, skip it. If you have enough time remaining at the end of the exam, go back to it.
10. Be sure to answer ALL questions; any left unanswered will be scored as a wrong response.

- Questions that require critical thinking are seen throughout the certification examinations. This means that you will be problem-solving, using logic to select the best solution to problem situations presented.
  - For example: You know the definition of "triage," but you need to apply it to a given scenario posed to you in a multiple-choice question.

The following is an example of a critical thinking question:

You are employed at an OB/GYN practice. The physician has confirmed a suspected pregnancy of one of your husband's family relatives. The relative nervously lets you know that no one else knows about this office visit. The most appropriate response is:

A. "If someone asks, I'll only tell them you had an office appointment."
B. "Be assured in knowing that I don't discuss or share any patient information outside of the office."
C. "Trust me, I'll only tell my husband."
D. "This is such happy news, it should be shared."
E. "You should be very happy about this.

This question presents a situation in which you must decide the best way to respond. It is testing your ability to recognize your professional responsibility in ensuring that a patient's needs are appropriately met.

- When you believe you know material in a tab section . . . **Test yourself**! A CD icon has been inserted at the end of each tab or major section as a reminder.
- Last, but certainly not least, remember to relax! You've been studying hard and you know the answers. If you feel yourself tensing up during your examination, here's a little technique that works. Lick your lips and inhale quietly and slowly through your mouth. Concentrate on that cool sensation you get—it's relaxing. Now get back to the examination with a more relaxed and open mind. You may want to practice this technique in attempting a successful outcome while using the enclosed CD to create simulated examinations. You know the answers; use your knowledge and logical thinking!

Examinations and Test Application Processing

AMT

1. Applications must be completed and submitted with required documentation and a certified check.
2. The AMT processes the application, then notifies the applicant to select a computer testing agency from an approved list.
3. The applicant contacts the agency to arrange a convenient test date, and time. MA education institutions also may serve as computer testing centers upon AMT approval.
4. Application questions? Visit www.amt1.com or phone 1-800-275-1268.

AAMA

1. Applications must be completed and submitted with required documentation and a certified check.
2. The AAMA processes the application, then sends a scheduling permit to the applicant.
3. Applicant must contact approved Prometric Test Center (www.prometric.com) to schedule the examination within 30 days of receipt.
4. Effective January 1, 2010, an applicant will be limited to three attempts to obtain their credential.
5. Application questions? E-mail certification@aama-ntl.org or phone 1-800-228-2262 or1-312-899-1500.

AMT National Examinations to Earn RMA/CMAS

- Examinations are timed.
- Each consists of 210 multiple-choice questions with four choices for each question (A through D).
- Each question is weighted in value ($\frac{1}{4}$ point to 1 full point).
- Minimum score of 70 is required to pass; this is scaled.
- Applicants will know immediately upon completion of computerized examination if they have earned RMA/CMAS credential.

Content Outline of RMA Examination

Approximately 41%: General Knowledge
Anatomy and physiology (A&P), medical terminology, medical law and ethics, human relations, patient education.

Approximately 24%: Administrative Knowledge
Insurance, financial and bookkeeping, medical receptionist/secretarial/clerical.

Approximately 35%: Clinical Knowledge
Asepsis, sterilization, instruments, vital signs and mensurations, physical examinations, clinical pharmacology, minor surgery, therapeutic modalities, laboratory procedures, EKGs, first aid.

Source: The Registered Medical Assistant Candidate Handbook, AMT

Content Outline of CMAS Examination

13%: MA Foundations
Terminology, A&P, law and ethics, professionalism.

8%: Basic Clinical
Patient history, charting, vital signs, asepsis, examination preparation, office emergencies, pharmacology.

10%: Clerical
Scheduling, communication, patient information, community resources.

14%: Records Management
Systems, procedures, confidentiality.

17%: Insurance Processing, Coding, Billing

17%: Financial Management
Bookkeeping and office accounting, banking, payroll.

7%: Information Processing
Computing and its applications.

14%: Office Management
Communications, business organization, human resources, safety, supplies and equipment, physical site, risk management, quality assurance.

Source: The Certified Medical Administrative Specialist Candidate Handbook, AMT

AAMA National Examination To Earn CMA Credential

- Examination is timed.
- As of January 2009, examination consists of 200 questions with five choices to each question (A through E); 20 of the 200 are "pretesting questions" (preselected, not scored).
- Applicant will receive immediate unofficial pass/fail result and will formally know if they have earned the CMA credential approximately 12 weeks after completing the examination.

Content Outline of CMA Examination

Approximately 33%: General
Medical terminology, A&P, psychology, professionalism, communication, medicolegal guidelines and requirements.

Approximately 33%: Administrative
Data entry, office equipment, computer concepts, records management, screening and processing mail, scheduling and monitoring appointments, resource information and community services, office environment, policies and procedures, practice finances, accounting and banking.

Approximately 33%: Clinical
Infection control, treatment area, patient preparation and assisting physician, patient history interview, collecting and processing specimens,

diagnostic testing, preparing and administering medications, emergencies, first aid, nutrition.

Source: Resource Library at AAMA-ntl.org

Tools

Additional Common Abbreviations

ABC	airway, breathing, circulation
AD	Alzheimer's disease
AK	above the knee
AKA	above the knee amputation
ama	against medical advice
ANS	autonomic nervous system
A&P	anterior and posterior; auscultation and percussion
ARDS	adult respiratory distress syndrome
ARF	acute respiratory failure; acute renal failure; acute rheumatic fever
A&W	alive and well
BK	below the knee
BP, B/P	blood pressure
BPM	beats per minute
BRAT	bananas, rice, applesauce, toast (BRAT diet)
BSA	body surface area
CF	cystic fibrosis
CNS	central nervous system
C/O,	complains of
CTS	carpal tunnel syndrome
D&C	dilation and curettage
DRG	diagnostic related group
EMS	emergency medical services
ER	emergency room
FUO	fever of undetermined origin
FYI	for your information
H&H, H/H	hematocrit and hemoglobin
HBP	high blood pressure
HR	heart rate
HRT	hormone replacement therapy

ICU	intensive care unit
I&D	incision and drainage
ins	insurance
IVP	intravenous pyelogram
L&A	light and accommodation
LBP	low blood pressure
LLQ	lower left quadrant
LMP	last menstrual period
LUQ	left upper quadrant
L&W	living and well
MA	mental age
OTC	over the counter
PNS	peripheral nervous system
REM	rapid eye movement
RLQ	right lower quadrant
RUQ	right upper quadrant
SIDS	sudden infant death syndrome
TC	throat culture; telephone call
TIA	transient ischemic attack
TPR	temperature, pulse, respiration
UC	urine culture
UTI	urinary tract infection

Study Tools

Use the following forms to help you create and track a study plan.

Examination Study Plan/Record

Examination Date:____________________

Week of____________________ (circle one) Study: First Second Third Fourth Fifth Sixth Last Again

Tab 2: Front Office	**Monday**	**Tuesday**	**Wednesday**	**Thursday**	**Friday**	**Saturday**	**Sunday**
Example: Office equipment & mail	*Read*	*Reviewed*	*Quizzed*			*Reviewed again*	

Examination Date:____________________

Week of____________________ (circle one) Study: First Second Third Fourth Fifth Sixth Last Again

Tab 3: Law & Ethics	Monday	Tuesday	Wednesday	Thursday	Friday	Saturday	Sunday

Examination Date:______________________

Week of__________________ (circle one) Study: First Second Third Fourth Fifth Sixth Last Again

Tab 4: Terminology/ Anatomy & Physiology	**Monday**	**Tuesday**	**Wednesday**	**Thursday**	**Friday**	**Saturday**	**Sunday**

Examination Date:____________________

Week of____________________ (circle one) Study: First Second Third Fourth Fifth Sixth Last Again

Tab 5: Clinical	Monday	Tuesday	Wednesday	Thursday	Friday	Saturday	Sunday

Examination Date:____________________

Week of__________________ (circle one) Study: First Second Third Fourth Fifth Sixth Last Again

Tab 6: Pharmacology	**Monday**	**Tuesday**	**Wednesday**	**Thursday**	**Friday**	**Saturday**	**Sunday**

Examination Date:____________________

Week of__________________ (circle one) Study: First Second Third Fourth Fifth Sixth Last Again

Tab 7: Laboratory	**Monday**	**Tuesday**	**Wednesday**	**Thursday**	**Friday**	**Saturday**	**Sunday**

Examination Date:____________________

Week of____________________ (circle one) Study: First Second Third Fourth Fifth Sixth Last Again

Tab 8: Psychology & Communication	**Monday**	**Tuesday**	**Wednesday**	**Thursday**	**Friday**	**Saturday**	**Sunday**

Examination Preparation Progress Record

Use this log to keep track of your progress toward examination readiness.

Suggested Keys for Marking Mastery Level		
No mark = Not yet studied	**M** = Mastered (100% correct)	**K** = Knowledgeable (80% or more correct)
P = Passing grade (75% correct)	**I** = Improvement needed (60% or less correct)	

Tab 2: Front Office	Mastery Level	Self-Test Scores			
Subject Area		1	2	3	4

Tab 3: Law & Ethics	Mastery Level	Self-Test Scores			
Subject Area		1	2	3	4

Tab 4: Term/A & P	**Mastery Level**	**Self-Test Scores**			
Subject Area		1	2	3	4

Tab 5: Clinical	**Mastery Level**	**Self-Test Scores**			
Subject Area		1	2	3	4

Tab 6: Pharm	**Mastery Level**	**Self-Test Scores**			
Subject Area		1	2	3	4

Tab 7: Lab	Mastery Level	Self-Test Scores			
Subject Area		1	2	3	4

Tab 8: Psych/Comm	Mastery Level	Self-Test Scores			
Subject Area		1	2	3	4

Schedule Planner/Organizer Month ________

Sunday	Monday	Tuesday	Wednesday	Thursday	Friday	Saturday

Schedule Planner/Organizer Month ________

Sunday	Monday	Tuesday	Wednesday	Thursday	Friday	Saturday

Schedule Planner/Organizer Month ________

Sunday	Monday	Tuesday	Wednesday	Thursday	Friday	Saturday

Schedule Planner/Organizer Month ________

Sunday	Monday	Tuesday	Wednesday	Thursday	Friday	Saturday

Notes

Preparation for the Day

Safety Hazards: Area rugs, electrical cords, traffic flow.
Ergonomics: Space, furnishings, equipment designed for effectiveness, safety, comfort.
Collating Records: Usually done day before; organizing records by content needs and the order in which patients are seen.

Office Equipment

Computer

Password: Each employee has own; to track employee computer activity.
ROM (read-only memory): Permanent, unchangeable basic operating instructions.
RAM (random access memory): Temporary memory; in use while using software; may be saved to drives.
CPU (central processing unit): Computer's "brain," processes data.
Modem: Communicating through phone lines to connect computers.
Bit: Smallest unit of info inside computer; either a 0 or 1.
Byte: Unit of data having 8 bits (binary digits).
Megabyte (MB): 1 Million bytes.
Gigabyte (GB): 1 Billion bytes (1,000 MB).
Terabyte (TB): 1,000 GB.
Networking: Computers are linked together to share information in office setting.
Purging: Removing unnecessary old data from hard drive or disk drive.
Software: Installed program that enables computer to perform specific tasks.
Menu: Displays choices of available functions.
CD-RP: One-time recordable CD to store data.
CD-RW: Recordable CD that stores data and allows numerous rewrites.
Flash (jump) drive: Portable device; 2 or more GB capacity for files; plugs into USB computer port.
Input device: Keyboard, mouse.

Output device: Printer, monitor.
Hard copy: Printout of document seen on monitor.

- **Scanner**: Converts hard copy into electronic format to be read by computer.
- **Laser printer**: Gives highest quality (resolution) to printed hard copy; ↑ $.
- **Fax (facsimile)**: Sends hard copies of (medical records, business documents); located in area inaccessible to public; maintains confidentiality.
- **Copier**: Duplicates hard copy.

Your Notes

Sending and Receiving Mail

Annotating: Underlining significant words, highlights key points.
Postage meter: Cancels stamp, saves steps in post office mail processing.
Physician's personal mail: Place unopened mail on physician's desk in easily visible area (top of day's charts).

First Class Mail

- Weighs 13 oz or ↓.
- 108 inches or ↓ in combined length and widest area width.
- 1- to 3-day delivery.
- Postcards, no. 10-size envelopes, green diamond-bordered envelopes.

Priority Mail: Same as first class, ↑ 13 oz and 70 lbs. or ↓.
Parcel Post: 70 lbs or ↓; 130 inches in combined length and widest area width; 2- to 9-day delivery; books, catalogues, general merchandise.
Certified Mail: The words printed on paper have ↑ value (contracts, birth certificates, etc.).
Registered Mail: Has a ↑ $ value to item being sent (jewels, medications, etc.).
Express Mail: If sent by 5 pm, then received by next day; up to 70 lbs; proof of delivery; insured up to $100.
Special Delivery: Delivery ASAP once mail reaches local post office for final delivery.

Medical Records

Record ownership: Physician owns record material; patient owns information in the record.
Used to provide:

- Best medical care.
- Statistics.
- Liability case defense (good documentation = good risk management).
- Quality of treatment assessment.

Record retention: 7–10 years for adults; 7–10 years from reaching age of majority for minors.
Active files: Patient seen within 6 months to 3 years (dependent on practice specialty).
Inactive files: Patient not seen within 6 months to 3 years.
Closed files: Patient not expected to return (moving, age limit in pediatrics, death).
Release of records with authorization: Send copies only to designated physician.
Release of records without authorization: Life-threatening circumstance (unconscious).
Error correction: Medical/accounting records.

- Draw line through error.
- Write correct data above/below error; date, time, initial.
- Do not attempt to erase or use correction fluid/tape; all medical records are legal documents.

POMR record organization: Problem-Oriented Medical Record.

- Problems are numbered.
- Has database: Demographics, profile history, cc (chief complaint), case conceptualization, past assessments and test results; treatment plan: procedures, medications, instructions; progress notes: continuous care notes.

SOAP: Form of documentation (subjective/objective/assessment/plan).

- **Subjective**: Symptoms not seen, heard, measured; given by patient.
- **Objective**: Signs read in test results, heard, measured, observed.
- **Assessment**: Findings, combine subjective/objective info into probable diagnosis.
- **Plan**: Treatment based on diagnosis: Medication, further tests, education, therapy, etc.

SOMR record organization: Source-Oriented Medical Record.

- Record is divided in sections: Laboratory, progress notes, physical examinations (PEs), consultation reports, etc.
- In chronological order, most recent is on top in each section.

Filing Systems

- **Direct filing**: Alphabetic.
  - First indexing unit: Last name (surname).
  - Second indexing unit: First name.
  - Third indexing unit: Middle initial or name.
  - Fourth indexing unit: Titles, suffixes (Jr., Dr., Atty., etc.) .
- **Indirect filing**: Numerical; in large clinics, hospitals; provides highest confidentiality; uses terminal digit—filing order is read from right to left.
- **Color coding**: Easy retrieval; ↓ misfiles.
- **Subjective**: Topics arranged alphabetically.
- **Tickler**: Chronological file; date and time reminder to perform tasks.
- **Electronic**: EHR (electronic health record) software to create and use records; goal is paperless office.

Record Filing Procedures

- **Inspecting:** Make sure physician indicated that the chart was reviewed and required actions were done.
- **Indexing:** Determines where each document needs to be filed within chart.
- **Coding:** Highlight name/subject of document.
- **Sorting:** Use alphabetical method to subdivide documents.
- **Storing:** Document storage; placed in proper record, in proper section of record, in proper chronological order.

Your Notes

Scheduling

Physician preference: First consideration in creating practice scheduling system

Matrix: Blocked-off time slots for not scheduling appointments (office visits; OVs).

- Completed before scheduling any appointments.

Buffer times: Time slots unfilled until it is present day in office.

- More needed Mondays and Fridays.

Missed OVs: Document in medical record and make notation in day's schedule planner.

Cancellations: Document in medical record and make notation in day's schedule planner.

Open hours (tidal)	• First come, first served. • Common scheduling format in urgent care centers.
Wave	• Usually see four patients per hour. • All scheduled for top of hour, seen in order of arrival.
Modified wave	• In 1-hour frame; two patients given own specific time, two told to arrive at same time (e.g., 10:30).
Clustering	• Same type of OV all scheduled in same block (certain day, am or pm). • ↑ Efficiency and speed.
Double booking	• Two or more patients scheduled with same physician at same time, overbooking. • Not good schedule planning; causes many delays.
Stream (time specified)	• Each patient given own specific time. • Most common method of scheduling.

Health Care Coverage

Allowed charge: Maximum $ insurance carrier will cover for a provided service.

Assignment of benefits: authorizes insurance company to pay physician directly.

Beneficiary: Eligible person named by subscriber to receive insurance benefits.

Birthday rule: Determines which insurance is billed first if individual is beneficiary of more than one policy.

Capitation: Fixed $ amount paid by insurance to physician 1 to 2 times per month for each enrolled patient; number of OVs and types of service given patient do not matter.

Coordination of benefits: Limits benefits to 100% of cost of service when there is more than one insurance used for coverage.

DRG (diagnosis-related group): Services provided are related to diagnosis for hospital inpatients.

Electronic claims: Preferred method of claim submission; reduces time in mailing and claim processing.

Fee profile: A given physician's usual charges for various procedures compiled over time.

Fee schedule: Preset $ an insurance company allows for each service/procedure (e.g., physician charges $75 for 99213, insurance fee schedule allows $68 for 99213).

Fiscal agent: Company that processes insurance claims on behalf of health insurance; used by Medicare and Medicaid in each state.

NonPAR (non-participating physician): Expects full payment for billed services.

PAR (participating/member) member: Agrees to accept the allowed charge as 100% payment; physician writes off difference between charged and allowed charge.

Preauthorization: Approval from insurance company for service due to medical necessity.

Precertification: Process used with insurance company, determines coverage for specific service.

Premium: Dollar amount paid (by patient and/or employer) for insurance coverage.

- **Lowers cost of premium:**

  1. Deductible: Out-of-pocket $ before insurance makes payment.
  2. Copayment: Set amount patient pays for each office visit ($10, $15).
  3. Coinsurance: Percentage that patient pays for each office visit (usually 20%).

Professional courtesy: Reduction or free service to professional associate.

RA (Remittance Advice): EOB (Explanation Of Benefits); sent by insurance carrier; gives breakdown of benefit amounts for services billed.

RBRVS (Resource-Based Relative Value Scale): Used by Medicare, determines allowed charges; $ amounts vary geographically.

Release of information consent: Patient signs in order for physician to release date of service information to insurance for claim processing.

Rider: Addition made to an insurance policy; usually exclusions for pre-existing chronic conditions and/or procedures for a specific time (e.g., first 6 months).

Subscriber/policyholder: Primary person covered by insurance.

UCR: Used to determine payable insurance benefits.

- **U:** Usual fees physician charges for procedure.
- **C:** Customary fees charged by physicians in the same geographic area and specialty.
- **R:** Reasonable fees when the usual procedure is more complicated.

Utilization review: Examination of services provided; performed by unaffiliated group to determine medical necessity.

Third-party payer (administrator): Usually the paying insurance carrier.

Your Notes

Insurance Types and Health Plans

Type	Description
Major medical (catastrophic insurance)	Assists in paying ↑ $ for unexpected medical expenses (hospitalizations); usually has a ↑ deductible
Liability	Homeowner, business, auto insurance if injury occurs on site or in auto
Life	Pays a beneficiary set $ amount in case of policyholder death
Worker's Compensation	Medical and disability insurance coverage for employee death, injury, illness on the job or due to job; physician sends First Report of Occupational Injury within 72 hours of patient's first visit
Self-insured employer	Employer has staffed health facility on site to cover employee needs; drug testing, physical examinations, special job-related testing
Group	Offered by employers to employee groups; low premiums; good benefits; all employees may join in lieu of PE (physical examination)
Individual	Coverage purchased by individual; requires passing PE to qualify; ↑ premium cost; **Medigap, Crossover**: supplemental policy purchased by individual to pay Medicare deductibles and 20% co-pays
Indemnity	Specific $ paid for each service; patient pays any remaining $ due; works on a "fee for service" basis
Government	**Medicare**: Federal government • Part A: Automatic enrollment, inpatient coverage • Part B: Voluntary enrollment, yearly deductible, monthly premium due • Part C: Medicare managed care plans; replace Part A and B • Part D: Prescription (Rx) plans

	Medicaid: Title XIX; for medically indigent; federal and state funded; last health care coverage to bill if there is other coverage; automatic accepting of assignment and payment in full if patient treated; cannot bill patient for covered services **Medi/Medi**: Used to describe patient with Medicare and Medicaid **Tricare**: Covers families of military active personnel and retirees; three choices of health benefits: 1. Prime: HMO 2. Extra: Managed care network 3. Standard: Fee-for-service plan **CHAMPVA**: Covers families of veterans with total, permanent service-related disabilities and those who died in line of duty
Managed care	**HMO**: Federal government requires this option offered by employers **PPO**: Physician group contracts with insurer; not prepaid

Coding

CPT: Current Procedural Terminology

Developed by the American Medical Association (AMA); referred to as Level I codes; used for coding services provided by health professionals, supplies, equipment.

Six ways to begin looking in alphabetic index for code:

- Procedure or service performed (incisions, arthroscopy, etc.).
- Anatomic: Site, organ.
- Condition: Lesions, adhesions, tumors, etc.
- Synonym: Throat/pharynx, cancer/carcinoma, heart/cardiac, etc.
- Eponym: Under proper names of their inventors, discoverers (e.g., Colles fracture).
- Abbreviation: EEG, EKG, MRI, etc.

Six Numeric Sections of CPT Manual

Section	Description
Evaluation and management (E&M)	99201–99499 Three main components: **History** (HPI, PFSH: patient family social history) **Examination** ROS (review of systems)–one or more body systems one or more body systems) **Decision making** (straightforward to highly complex) Three contributing components: **Time, counseling, coordination of care**
Anesthesiology	00100–01999, 99100–99140
Surgery (largest section)	10040–69990
Radiology	70010–79999
Pathology and laboratory	80049–89399
Medicine (except anesthesiology)	90281–99199

Consultation: Provided by physician when advice/opinion is sought by another physician.

Down code: Insurance carrier finds irregularity with claim submitted; result is ↓ $ reimbursed.

Established patient: Has received service within past 3 years.

New patient: Has not received service in past 3 years from physician or their group.

Referral: When one physician sends patient to another physician to treat patient for problem/illness.

Unbundling: Using more than one CPT code in place of available single code to identify procedure.

Up code: Provider purposely submits claim coded for ↑ $ reimbursement without proper documentation.

HCPCS: Level II

- Developed by HCFA (now Centers for Medicare and Medicaid Services; CMS).
- Procedure coding; **national codes.**
- Used for laboratory, pathology, pharmaceutical, equipment, and transportation services provided to patients under government-funded health care.
- Alphanumeric: Begin with one letter, A through V.

HCPCS: Level III

- Used on a statewide basis; **local codes.**
- Providers can report developing trends in a particular state.
- **WXYZ codes.**

ICD: International Classification of Disease

- Developed by WHO (World Health Organization); morbidity coding; used for established diagnosis/conditions.

Volume I

- Tabular (numeric).
- Category, three digits; subcategory, four digits; subclassification, five digits.
- Each additional digit provides more specific description of disease/condition.

Volume II

- Alphabetical.
- Contains hypertension table, neoplasm table, drugs and chemicals table.

Special Codes

- E code: External cause of injury/illness; supplement to primary code.
- V code: Influences health status; example PE (physical examination), pregnancy, family history; may be the primary code.

Billing and Fee Collection

Cycle Billing

- Bills patient at same time each month according to first letter of last name (e.g., patients with last name beginning with A through F billed the 10th of each month).

Balance Billing

- Patient billed for difference between charge and insurance payment.

Types of Payment

- At time of service.
- Bill with credit extension.
- Insurance (third party).
- Outside collection agency.

Credit Policy of Office

- Payment due dates.
- Payment due at time of service.
- Collection procedures including use of agency.
- Participating insurance companies and accepting assignment.

Age Analysis

- Outstanding remaining debt is aged from previous dates of service still owed to practice.

Total Account Receivable	Amount that is 1–3 months old	Amount that is 4–6 months old	Amount that is 6–9 months old	Amount that is 10–12 months old
$425.00	$75.00	$280.00	$70.00	$0.00

Collection Agency

- Billing of last resort.
- Agency keeps 40%–60% of collected amount.
- Do not send bills or discuss account with patient after submitting account to agency.

Bookkeeping/Accounting

Bookkeeping: Detailed Recorded Part of Accounting

Adjustment: $ written off, the office will not collect it.

- Usually result of participating with insurance.
- Difference between amount charged and amount allowed by insurance.

Assets: Possessions of value—office equipment, inventory, prepaid payables (rent).
Balance: $ difference between the fee charged and the payment made toward it.
Balance sheet: For specific date needed, shows total assets, liabilities, and capital of business.
Charge: Fee incurred for a provided service.
Credit: Payment made toward a debit.
Credit balance: Payments made from different sources that result in overpayment.
Debit: Debt, money owed for services charged.
Double entry: CPAs use.

- Checks and balances; assets = liabilities + capital.

Liabilities: $ owed to others (rent, phone, equipment leases, etc.).
Posting: The act of recording information.

- Noting payment in day sheet, account ledger, etc.

Single Entry System: Simplest; simple summaries.

- Difficult to find errors.

Superbill, Encounter Form, Charge Slip, Statement: May be used to bill insurance.

- Contains ICDs, CPTs, patient insurance information, MD information and signature.

Transaction: Any exchange, such as services provided for a fee.

Accounting: Summarized Bookkeeping Transactions

Account ledger: Each patient has one.

- All of patient's financial transactions are recorded here.

Accounts payable: $ owed by practice (provider).
Accounts receivable: $ owed to the practice (provider).
Account receivable control: Total $ owed to practice by close of business day.
Accrual basis: When items sold, but may not be paid for, it is considered income.
Cash basis: Used by medical offices; charges entered as income when payment received.
Disbursement record: Part of accounts payable.

- Shows each amount paid out, date and check number, category of payment office supplies, medical supplies, etc.).

General journal (day sheet): Detailed chronologic record of services given, charges, and receipts.

- Information is first recorded here.

Payroll record: Part of accounts payable.

- Kept separate from other payables.

Petty Cash: Part of accounts payable.

- Pays for minor unexpected expenditures.

Banking

ABA number: Upper right of check.

- Identifies exact bank location of check origin.

Bank draft: Check written by bank against its funds in another bank.
Bank statements: Record of all checkbook financial transactions.

- Displays processed deposits and checks, interest earned, and service charges over a specific time frame: first of month to last day of given month.

Cashier's check: Treasurer's check; bank's own check and signed by bank representative.
Certified check: Payer's own check, officially stamped by bank.

- Guarantees availability of funds by setting amount in account aside.

Checkbook: Receipts are recorded and deposited here.

- Bills (accounts payable) are made from here and recorded here.

Limited check: Has a time limit (90 days) or preprinted for maximum amount limit.
MICR code: Magnetic ink character recognition.

- Magnetic printed code across bottom of check.
- Used by bank for sorting checks.

Overdraft (NSF): Nonsufficient funds (bounced check).

- Too ↓ $ in account to cover check amount.

Payee: Person, practice, or company to whom the check is written (payable).
Payer: Person who signs the check to release $ to the payee.
Power of attorney: Grants legal right to handle financial matters of another's account.
Reconciliation: Balancing a checkbook with the bank statement.

- Start with bank statement $ balance; then add deposits not seen on statement; then subtract outstanding checks not seen on statement; the remaining $ should be the checkbook balance.

Third-party check: Written by unknown party to payee.

- Only accept insurance checks with limited endorsement to practice.

Traveler's check: To use where personal checks may not be accepted.

- Purchased from bank for small fee.

Types of endorsements

- **Blank**: Most common, signature only.
- **Restrictive**: "For deposit only" stamped on check back.
- **Limited (special)**: "Pay to the order of" followed by signature of patient paying.
- **Qualified**: "Without recourse" used by lawyers accepting checks by clients.

Voucher check: With detachable part giving payee additional information (i.e., payroll checks).

Supply Inventory and Ordering

Invoice: May be included with delivered items; displays amount due for each item.
Packing slip: Included with product delivery; describes items enclosed.
Statement: Bill for all invoices of items delivered during one month.

Office Management

Manuals

Office Policy content:

- Mission statement.
- Office's organizational chart.
- Position interviewing, hiring, firing.
- Sick leave, vacation.
- Personnel evaluations.
- Dress code.
- Staff meetings.

- Work flow.
- Office maintenance.

Procedure content:

- Job descriptions (clinical MA, LPN, receptionist, etc.).
- Step-by-step guide for each procedure in a given position.

Payroll and Forms

Gross: Total amount earned in pay period, before deductions are made.
Net: Earned income after deductions are made.
Salary: Fixed amount paid to employee regardless of hours worked in pay period.
Wages: $ paid per hour, in a 40-hour week.

- More than 40 hours per week: 1.5 times hourly wage for overtime hours.

EIN (Employer tax ID number): Each employer must have for reporting federal taxes.
Employment forms

- **W2**: Federal tax form given employees in January; previous year's wage detail.
- **W4**: Employees withholding allowance certificate; completed prior to first pay period; number of tax exemptions are noted here.

FICA (Federal Insurance and Contribution Act): Social Security and Medicare percentage of income withheld from employee paychecks.

- **Deposit Requirements**: Done by employer each month to federal deposit account in a federal reserve or authorized bank.
- $ amount: Federal tax withheld plus two times the FICA tax withheld.

Form 940 FUTA (Federal Unemployment Tax Act): Paid annually to IRS.

- Percentage of employee's paycheck paid by employer toward unemployment fund, not deducted from employee gross income.

Form 941: Employer's quarterly federal tax return to report federal income tax and FICA taxes withheld from employee paychecks; due within 1 month after each quarter—April 30, July 31, October 31, January 31.

Financial Summaries

Practice Management Reports

Accounts receivable ratio: Measures speed at which outstanding balances are paid.
Cash flow statement: Displays balance at start date and end date with all expenses and income receipts within time frame.
Collection ratio: Measures effectiveness of office billing system (e.g., 97% of billed amount is paid).
Disbursements journal: Summary of accounts paid out.
Statement of income and expense (profit and loss): Summary of all income and expenses for a time period.
Trial balance: Checks accuracy of accounts.

- Accounts receivable control should match total of all patient's accounts receivable ledgers.

Office Meetings

Meeting agenda: Orderly listing of items to be discussed at formal meeting.
Meeting minutes: Official record of previous meeting.

- Must be approved by motion.
- Contents are: name of committee; date, time, type of meeting; members present; items of business discussed (no summaries); motions made, approved, rejected; adjournment time, next meeting date if any.

Office Equipment

Maintenance agreements: Made for periodic upkeep (cleaning) of computers, copiers, fax machines, typewriters, etc.
Replacement: Usually in maintenance agreement.

- Office pays for replaced part, not labor.

Warranty: Sent to manufacturer upon receipt of equipment.

- Ensures replacement of defective parts and equipment.
- Usually has replacement period up to 1 year from purchase.

Your Notes

Think you got all that?

Test yourself using your enclosed CD-ROM!

Notes

Laws

Society's mandated rules; governmental punishment for failure to observe.

Source of Law: Three Branches of Government

Legislative (Congress): Passes law.
Executive: Administers law.
Judicial: Interprets and enforces law.

Main Areas of Law

1. **Criminal:** Crimes committed against society, individual, or property.

Government prosecutes, and if found guilty, result is imprisonment or fine.

2. **Civil:** Crimes committed against individual or property by an individual/organization.

Individual/group prosecutes, and if found guilty, result is monetary compensation.

Types of Civil Law

1. Tort

Accidental/intentional wrongful act by someone against another/property.
Negligence (common tort): Failure to perform professional duties prudently, according to accepted standard of care.
Forms of negligence:

- **Nonfeasance:** Failure to act when duty indicated; results in injury to another.
- **Misfeasance:** Improper performance of act; results in injury to another.
- **Malfeasance:** Committing improper (illegal) act; results in injury to another.

- **Malpractice ("professional negligence")**: Professional misconduct, lack of skill, wrongful practice; results in injury to another.
  - **Res ipsa loquitur**: "The thing speaks for itself"; negligence is obvious and the event could not have occurred without negligence.
  - **Respondeat superior**: "Let the master answer"; provider may not be directly responsible, but is responsible for negligence of employees.

- **The "Four Ds" of malpractice are**:
  1. **Duty**: The provider and patient relationship was established.
  2. **Dereliction**: The provider neglected a professional obligation to act or acted improperly.
  3. **Direct cause**: Negative outcome was a direct result from provider's actions or failure to act.
  4. **Damages**: A negative act resulted in the patient sustaining harm.

2. **Contract**

- Dealing with created agreements made that are enforceable obligations and rights.
  1. **Express contract**: Verbalized agreement between two parties; oral or written.
  2. **Implied contract**: Result of actions (provider treats a patient).

Consent: An agreement between legally capable parties, legal intent is made; an offer is made and accepted, and transaction (service, payment) is made.

Quid pro quo: Something for something, i.e., service for payment.

Consenter: Competent adult, emancipated minor (under 18), minors in armed forces, minor parent with custody, minors seeking sexually related treatment.

- **Informed**: Patient's right to know before agreeing to treatment, procedures, care.
- **Uninformed**: Patient gives permission without full understanding.

Advance directives: Document states patients' wishes should they become incapable of making own decisions; signed and witnessed.

- **Living will**: Patient's wish to not have certain life-sustaining measures taken when prognosis is imminent death.

- **Durable power of attorney (health care):** Allows one to act on behalf of patient to determine use of heroic/extraordinary measures.

3. **Administrative**

- Government agency enforced requirements and standards (i.e., FDA).
- **Some related to medical office operations are:**

OSHA (Occupational Safety and Health Administration): Regulates safety in workplace for employees and patients.
CLIA (Clinical Laboratory Improvement Amendments): Regulates laboratory testing standards for quality assurance.
IRS (Internal Revenue Service): Regulates payroll taxes.
DEA (Drug Enforcement Administration): Regulates provider registration and all handling of controlled substances (i.e., medications) in office.

Your Notes

Ambulatory Health Care Employee Credentials

Licensed

- Granted by individual states upon meeting requirements (passing **required** examination and paying fee) to legally practice within scope of field.
- Highest regulation; examples are:
  - MD (medical doctor), DO (doctor of osteopathy), RN (registered nurse), LPN (licensed practical nurse), LVN (licensed vocational nurse).

Reciprocity: License to practice granted when one state recognizes and accepts another state's licensing procedure.

License Revocation/Suspension

1. Convicted of a crime.
2. Guilty of unprofessional conduct (dishonesty, falsifying records).
3. Incapable professionally/personally (substance abuse, practicing outside trained scope).

Certification

- Granted by professional organization upon meeting requirements (passing examination and paying fee); examination is usually for national certification; examples are:
  - CMA (through American Association of Medical Assistants; medical assistant), RMA (through American Medical Technologists [AMT]; medical assistant), CMAS (through AMT; medical administrative specialist), MLT (medical laboratory technician), MT (medical technologist), CMT (medical transcriptionist), CCA (coding associate), CCS (coding specialist).

Licensed and/or Certified

- State regulation may require one or both for:

NP (nurse practitioner), PA (physician assistant).

Registration

- Granted by professional organization upon fee payment to become listed in a registry of field.

Types of Medical Practice

Solo practice: Owns practice; makes all decisions; retains all profits, costs, and liabilities.

Partnership: Written agreement; shared costs, liabilities, profits, decision making.

Group practice: Three or more providers; share costs, profits, decisions (usually primary care, one specialty, or multi-specialty group).

Professional Service Corporation: Various professionals (one or more providers, lawyers, etc.); fringes include profit sharing, pensions; individual liability; state law regulation.

Laws and Acts

Americans with Disabilities Act (ADA): Prohibits discrimination (with 15 or more employees) in employment practices; hiring, fringes, leaves, terminations. Public accommodations must be made architecturally and to practice policies.

Child Abuse Prevention and Treatment Act: State mandates for reporting of suspected child abuse and neglect; all professionally trained personnel working with children must report this.

Civil Rights Act: Governs all forms of discrimination among employees, supervisors, employers.

CLIA (Clinical Laboratory Improvement Act): Quality and complexity level regulations for hospital, private, and physician office laboratories (POLs); laboratory levels are either waived, moderately complex, or highly complex.

Controlled Substances Act: Initiated by DEA; narcotic/dangerous drug regulation in prescribing, dispensing, administering due to potential abuse.

Employee Retirement Income Security Act (ERISA): Protects/regulates employee pensions.

Equal Credit Opportunity Act: Ensures all patients are offered extended credit; denial of offer must be based on inability-to-pay rationale.

Equal Employment Opportunity Act (EEOA): Prohibits inquiry on job applications of race, color, sex, religion, national origin, medical history, arrest records, and past substance abuse.

Fair Credit Billing Act: Establishes time limits in billing complaints—patient has 60 days to complain; medical facility has 90 days to respond.

Fair Debt Collections Practices Act: Regulates debt collection practice; eliminates unfair practice.

Fair Labor Standards Act: Regulates employee wages and pay records, overtime pay, child labor.

Family and Medical Leave Act (FMLA): Applies if employed 1 year; allows leave without position loss up to 12 weeks in sites employing over 50 persons (i.e., birth, adoption; ill family member; own illness).

Federal wage garnishing law: Sets $ limits that can be attached to person's wages/property in order to pay large debt.

Good Samaritan law: Health care employee giving aid to non-paying individuals outside place of employment; employee protected from tort claims or liability.

Health Insurance Portability and Accountability Act (HIPAA): Provides national guidelines for health care privacy protection by:

- New job, increased chance of health insurance coverage—continuous or new.
- Ensures privacy of all health and identification information.
- Patient shared information is just for: treatment, payment, medical office operations.

Medical Practice Acts: Each state's statutes that govern practice of medicine (education, licensing and renewals, suspension and revocation of license).

Occupational Safety and Health Act (OSHA): Regulates employee safety from known hazards causing death/injury; **Material Safety Data Sheets (MSDS)** on hazardous products at site available to employees.

Patient's Bill of Rights: American Hospital Association (AHA) statement guaranteeing patient's certain rights (service, confidentiality, receipt of updated information regarding diagnosis, treatment, PE; receipt of all information regarding procedures, bill examination and understanding, etc.).

Patient Self-Determination Act: Requires written information regarding rights, medical decision making, and execution of advance directives be provided by health care worker.

Truth in Lending Act (Regulation Z): Signed agreement for full debt payment in over four payments; agreement also stipulates applied/non-applied finance charge.

Uniform Anatomical Gift Act: States that:

- Anyone of sound mind over 18 years of age may donate all or parts of their body after death.
- Time of death determined by provider unrelated to transplant/research.
- Provider cannot be sued upon acceptance of body parts with proper documents.

More Terms and Definitions

Arbitration

- A dispute between parties is settled by the judgment by an uninvolved third-party person (or group) mutually selected by disputing parties.

Battery

- Touching a person without a legally justifiable reason or nonconsensual that is considered to be harmful or offensive.
- An intentional tort.

Confidentiality

- Major ethical area of concern for all health care professionals.
- Information is gained as a result of the physician-patient relationship.
- Referred to as privileged communication.
- Medical records: hard copy, electronic health records (EHR), and electronic medical records (EMR)—only medical staff may have access to these.
  - **Subpoena duces tecum:** Commands an individual to appear in court with a patient's medical record or other pertinent documents for the court.
- Maintaining this is a component of professional work ethic.

Defamation

- False, malicious communication to third party; works to damage a person's reputation.

Defendant

- Action (i.e., lawsuit) is being brought against this party.

Emancipated Minor

- Under the age of 18.
- Responsible for his/her own debts.

Libel

- Defamatory communication that is written.

Moral

- Concern for ideas about right and wrong.

Plaintiff

- Party bringing the suit or claim to court.

Slander

- Defamatory communication that is verbal.

Standard of Care

- Care given by a sound and rational person in the same situation.

Ethics

- Moral guidelines, principles, code for behavior, felt to be right when reflected upon.
- Continued education in field of practice are contribution to community.

Medical Ethics

- Moral conduct of people in medical professions.
  1. Contributes to well-being of community.
  2. Responsibility to society is continuing field education.
  3. Every medical profession has a "code of ethics."
  4. The result(s) of failure to adhere to ethical standards are:
     - Negative reputation.
     - Certification or license suspension by licensing or certifying board.
     - Certification or license revocation by licensing or certifying board.

Your Notes

AMT American Medical Technologists Standards of Practice

Members of the AMT Registry must recognize their responsibilities, not only to their patients, but also to society, to other health care professionals, and to themselves. The following standards of practice are principles adopted by the AMT Board of Directors, which define the essence of honorable and ethical behavior for a health care professional.

1. While engaged in the Arts and Sciences, which constitute the practice of their profession, AMT professionals shall be dedicated to the provision of competent service.
2. The AMT professional shall place the welfare of the patient above all else.
3. The AMT professional understands the importance of thoroughness in the performance of duty, compassion with patients, and the importance of the tasks, which may be performed.
4. The AMT professional shall always seek to respect the rights of patients and of health care providers, and shall safeguard patient confidences.
5. The AMT professional will strive to increase his/her technical knowledge, shall continue to study, and apply scientific advanced in his/her specialty.
6. The AMT professional shall respect the law and will pledge to avoid dishonest, unethical, or illegal practices.
7. The AMT professional understands that he/she is not to make or offer a diagnosis or interpretation unless he/she is a duly licensed physician/dentist or unless asked by the attending physician/dentist.
8. The AMT professional shall protect and value the judgment of the attending physician or dentist, providing this does not conflict with the behavior necessary to carry out Standard Number 2 above.
9. The AMT professional recognizes that any personal wrongdoing is his/her responsibility. It is also the professional health care provider's obligation to report to the proper authorities any knowledge of professional abuse.
10. The AMT professional pledges personal honor and integrity to cooperate in the advancement and expansion, by every lawful means, of American Medical Technologists.

Source: AMT Web site (www.amt1.com)

AAMA Medical Assisting Code of Ethics

The Code of Ethics of the American Association of Medical Assistants (AAMA) shall set forth principles of ethical and moral conduct as they relate to the medical profession and the particular practice of medical assisting.

Members of AAMA dedicated to the conscientious pursuit of their profession, and thus desiring to merit the high regard of the entire medical profession and the respect of the general public which they serve, do pledge themselves to strive always to:

A. Render service with full respect for the dignity of humanity;
B. Respect confidential information obtained through employment unless legally authorized or required by responsible performance of duty to divulge such information;
C. Uphold the honor and high principles of the profession and accept its disciplines;
D. Seek to continually improve the knowledge and skills of medical assistants for the benefit of patients and professional colleagues;
E. Participate in additional service activities aimed toward improving the health and well-being of the community.

Source: AAMA Web site (www.aama-ntl.org)

Bioethics

Current biological technology; often life-and-death moral issues. Public makes choices; no laws govern that choice.

Think you got all that?

 **Test yourself using your enclosed CD-ROM!**

Notes

Directional Terminology

Term	Definition	Example of Usage
Left (L)	L side of patient's body	Stomach is to L of liver
Right (R)	R side of patient's body	"The R kidney is damaged."
Superior	Toward top of body	Shoulders are superior to hips
Inferior	Toward lower end of body	Stomach is inferior to heart
Anterior/ventral	Toward front of body	Nose is on anterior of head
Posterior/dorsal	Toward back of body	Heel is posterior to head
Caudad (caudal)	Toward tail	Neck is caudad to skull
Cephalad	Toward head	Neck is cephalad to tail
Medial	Toward midsagittal; away from side	Eyes are medial to ears
Lateral	Toward side; away from midsagittal	Eyes are lateral to nose
Distal	Away from point of origin; away from trunk or point of attachment	Hand is distal to elbow
Proximal	Closest to point of origin, toward trunk (position in a limb or appendage)	Joint is proximal to toenail
Visceral	Toward internal organ; away from outer wall	Organ covered with visceral layer of the membrane
Parietal	Toward wall; away from internal structures	Abdominal cavity lined with parietal peritoneal membranes
Deep	Toward inside of part; away from surface	Thigh muscles deep to skin

Continued

Term	Definition	Example of Usage
Superficial	Toward surface of part; away from inside	Skin is a superficial organ
Medullary	Refers to an inner region, or medulla	Medullary portion of organ, contains nerve tissue
Cortical	Refers to an outer region or cortex	This area produces hormones

Movement Terminology

Adduction: State of drawing toward middle.

Abduction: State of drawing away from middle.

Afferent: Send toward center; afferent nerves carry impulses to central nervous system (CNS).

Circumduction: Drawing an imaginary circle with body part (finger movement, arm movement).

Efferent: Send away from center; efferent nerves carry info away from CNS to muscles/glands.

Eversion: State of turning outward (turning wrists and ankles outward, away from body).

Extension: Limb moves into a straight position (straightening hand fingers).

Flexion: Movement in which a limb is bent (making a fist).

Inversion: State of turning inward.

Plantar flexion: Pointing toes downward.

Prone: Lying straight on one's front; face down.

Rotation: Turning on an axis (head turning side to side).

Supine: Lying straight on one's back, face up.

Common Prefixes and Suffixes

Prefix	Common Meaning	Suffix	Common Meaning
a, an	Without or absence of	ac, al, ar, ary	Pertaining to
ab	Away from	algia	Pain, suffering
ad, af, ap, as, at	Toward, in the direction of	apheresis	Removal
ana	Excessive	asthenia	Weakness
bi	Two, life	atresis	Absence of normal body opening
bin	Two by two	cal	Pertaining to
brady	Slow	capnia	Carbon dioxide
dia	Through, complete	cele	Hernia, protrusion
dys	Bad, difficult, painful	centesis	Surgical puncture to remove fluid
endo	Within	clasis, clast	Break
epi	Upon	coccus	Berry-shaped bacterium
eti	Cause	crine	Secrete
eu	Good, normal, well, easy	crit	To separate
ex, exo	Outside, outward	cyte	Cell
hemi	Half	desis	Surgical fixation, fusion
hyper	Excessive, increased	drome	Run, running
hypo	Deficient, decreased	eal	Pertaining to
inter	Between, among	ectasis	Stretching out, dilation, expansion
intra	Within, inside	ectomy	Surgical removal
meta	Change, after, beyond	emia	Blood condition
neo	New	emesis	Vomiting

Continued

Common Prefixes and Suffixes—cont'd

Prefix	Common Meaning	Suffix	Common Meaning
nulli	None	gen	Agent that causes or produces
pan	All, total	genesis	Origin, cause
para	Beside, beyond, around	genic	Producing, causing, originating
per	Through	gram	An instrument for recording, picture, record
peri	Surrounding	graphy	Process of producing a picture
poly	Many	ia	Diseased, abnormal condition
post	After	iasis, esis	Condition
pre	Before	iatry	Physician, treatment
sub	Under, less, below	ical, ial, ic, ior	Pertaining to
super, supra	Above, excessive	ictal	Seizure, attack
syn, sym	Together, joined	itis	Inflammation
tachy	Fast, rapid	lysis	Loosening, dissolution, separating
tetra	Four	malacia	Abnormal softening
tri	Three	megaly	Enlargement
		meter	Instrument used to measure
		metry	Measurement
		necrosis	Tissue death
		odynea	Pain
		oid	Resembling
		ologist	Specialist

More Suffixes

Suffix	Meaning	Suffix	Meaning
ology	The study of	plegia	Paralysis
oma	Tumor	pnea	Breathing
opia	Vision	poiesis	Formation
opsy	To view	ptosis	Drooping, sagging, prolapse
ory, ose, ous	Pertaining to	rrhage, rrhagia	Bleeding, bursting forth
osis	Abnormal condition	rrhaphy	Surgical suturing
ostomy	Surgically created opening	rrhea	Flow, discharge
otomy	Surgical incision	rrhexis	Rupture
oxia	Oxygen	sarcoma	Malignant tumor
paresis	Slight paralysis	schisis	Split, fissure
pathy	Disease	scope	Visual examine with instrument
penia	Abnormal reduction in number	scopy	Visual examination
pepsia	Digestion	sis	State of
pexy	Surgical fixation, suspension	spasm	Sudden involuntary muscle contraction
phagia	Eating, swallowing	stasis	Control, maintenance at a constant level
phobia	Abnormal fear or aversion to	stenosis	Abnormal tightening, narrowing
phonia	Sound, voice	tome	Instrument used to cut

Continued

More Suffixes—cont'd

Suffix	Meaning	Suffix	Meaning
physis	Growth	tripsy	Surgical crushing
plasia	Formation	trophy	Development
plasm	Formative material of cells	thorax	Chest
plasty	Surgical repair	uria	Urine, urination

Common Word Roots

Root	Meaning	Root	Meaning
carcin, cancer	Cancer	melan	Black
chrom	Color	neur	Nerve
cyan	Blue	onc	Tumor
cyt	Cell	organ	Organ
erythr	Red	path	Disease
gno	Knowledge	rhabd	Rod-shaped or striated (tissue)
hist	Tissue	sarc	Flesh, connective tissue
kary	Nucleus	somat	Body
lei	Smooth	viscer	Internal organs
leuk	White	xanth	Yellow
lip	Fat		

Your Notes

Directions and Body Planes

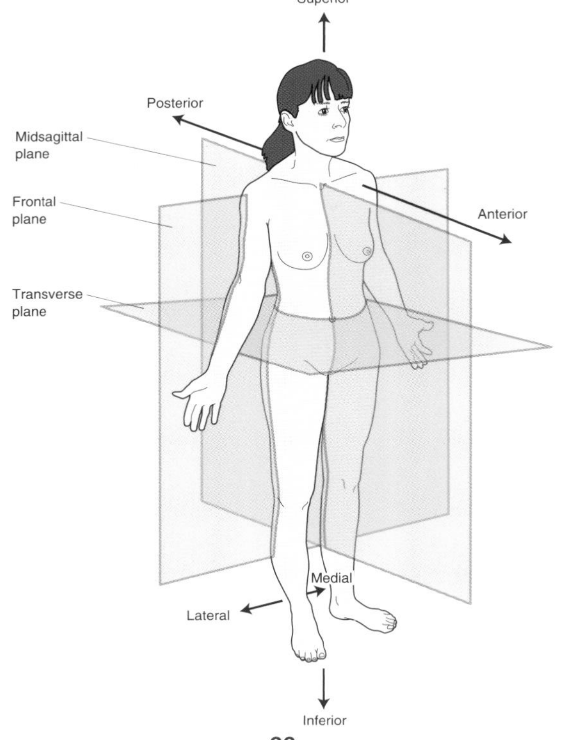

Body Cavities

Cranial cavity: Contains brain
Spinal cavity: Spinal cord; begins at brain stem
Thoracic cavity: Contains heart, lungs, large blood vessels; separated from abdomen by diaphragm
Abdominal cavity: Contains stomach, most of intestines, kidneys, liver, gallbladder, pancreas, spleen; separated from thoracic cavity by diaphragm and from pelvic cavity by imaginary line across top of hip bones
Pelvic cavity: Contains urinary bladder, rectum, male/female internal reproductive organs; separated from abdominal cavity by an imaginary line between the hip bones.

Nine Regions of the Abdominopelvic Cavity

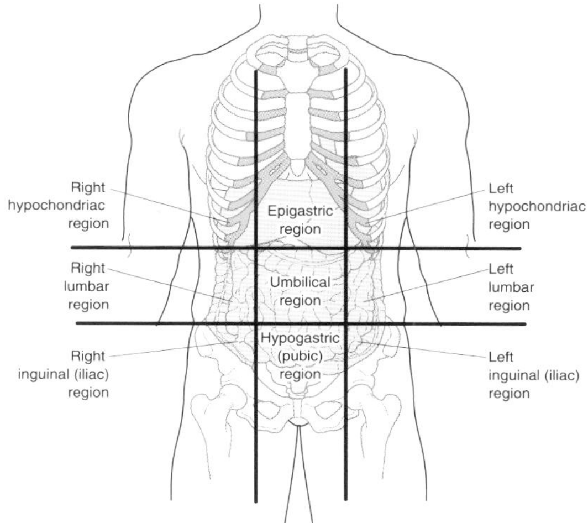

Organization

- **Homeostasis:** Equilibrium, maintaining a balance of the internal body (e.g., vital signs).
- **Atom:** Smallest chemical unit of matter.
- **Molecule:** Part of a compound that is a substance (e.g., H_2O).
- **Cell:** Basic unit of life, basic building block.
  - **Mitosis:** Cell division, one cell splits into two identical cells.
  - **Meiosis:** Cell division for organisms that sexually reproduce.

Active transport: Molecule movement from area of ↑ to ↓ concentration; requires cellular energy

Diffusion: Dissolved particles move from area of ↑ to ↓ concentration

Filtration: Liquids diffused through membranes only requiring mechanical pressure

Osmosis: Molecules of H_2O transported from an area of ↑ to ↓ concentration

Phagocytosis: Ingestion and digestion of substances by phagocytic cells; requires cellular energy

The Cell

- Golgi apparatus: Secretes mucus.
- Nucleus: Hold DNA-genetic code.
- Ribosomes: For protein synthesis.
- Mitochondria: Power plant, produce energy.
- Lysosomes: Aid in digestion.
- Centriole: Rod-shaped, begins cell division.
- Cytoplasm: Fluid filling the cell.
- Cilia: Hairlike; move particles across cell surface.
- Endoplasmic reticulum: Network of tubes to transport proteins, metabolism of lipids and carbohydrates.

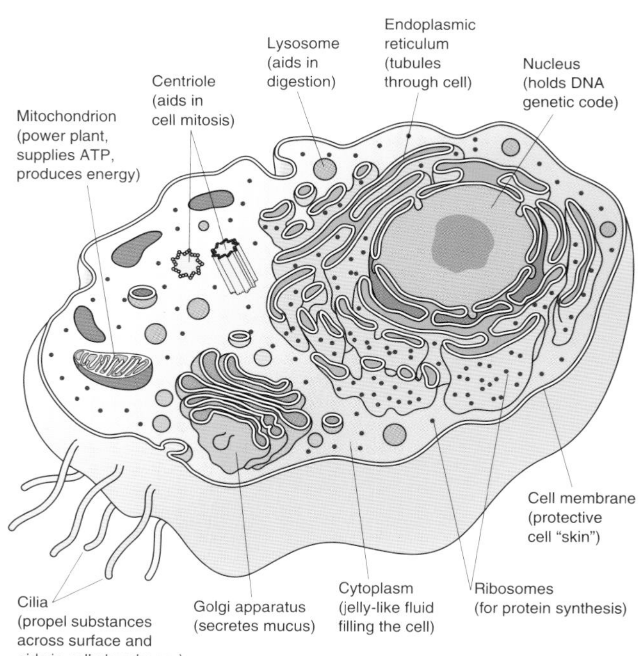
Endoplasmic
reticulum
(tubules
through cell)
Lysosome
(aids in
digestion)
Nucleus
(holds DNA
genetic code)
Centriole
(aids in
cell mitosis)
Mitochondrion
(power plant,
supplies ATP,
produces energy)
Cell membrane
(protective
cell "skin")
Cytoplasm
(jelly-like fluid
filling the cell)
Ribosomes
(for protein synthesis)
Cilia
(propel substances
across surface and
aids in cell absorbancy)
Golgi apparatus
(secretes mucus)

Tissue

- A grouping of cells that performs a specific function. Four types:

Tissue Type	Locations	Functions
Epithelial	Skin, tubes, ducts, some glands, lining cavities	Protection, absorption, secretions, excretions
Connective	Bones, tendons, muscle sheaths, blood	Supports, connects other tissues and structures
Muscle	**Three types:** striated, smooth, cardiac	Produces movement, contracts or shortens
Nerve	Neurons (cells) throughout body	Actively transmits impulses through networks

Organ

Group of tissues that serve a common purpose or function.

System

Group of organs working together to perform a specific function.

Your Notes

BODY SYSTEMS

Skeletal System

Functions	Cells, Tissues, Organs
1. Movement of body 2. Support of body (framework) 3. Attachment for muscle 4. Formation of RBCs in red bone marrow 5. Storage of calcium 6. Protection of internal organs	1. Joints 2. Ligaments 3. Cartilage 4. Bone (approximately 206)

Joint Classifications

Amphiarthrosis (slightly movable): Fibrocartilaginous disk between two bones, or a ligament uniting two bones.

Diarthrosis (freely movable): Bone ends joined by joint capsule lubricated by synovial fluid.

Synarthrosis (immovable): Two bones separated only by membrane (cranial sutures).

Motion Movement Groups

Ball and socket (enarthrosis): Hip.

Condyloid: All forms of angular movement except axial rotation—between metacarpals and phalanges.

Gliding (arthrodia): One bony surface slides on another.

Hinge (ginglymus): Synovial joint having only 1 forward and backward motion—elbow.

Pivot (trichoid): Permits rotation of bone.

Saddle: Opposing surfaces are reciprocally concavoconvex—between carpal and metacarpal of thumb.

Additional Information

Foramen: Hole in bone for passage of vessels or nerves.

Periosteum: Thick fibrous membrane, covers bone surface except articular cartilage.

Synovial fluid: Lubricating fluid of joint, bursae, and tendon sheaths.

Axial Skeleton: The Major Bones	Appendicular Skeleton
Cranium (skull): Seams are sutures **Frontal**: Forehead and eye sockets **Temporal**: Sides around ear and lower jaw **Parietal**: Sides above temporal and top **Occipital**: Back of head and skull base	**Upper Extremities** **Humerus**: Upper arm, **largest arm bone** **Radius**: Lower arm, on thumb side **Ulna**: Lower arm, on little finger side **Carpals**: Wrist bones **Metacarpals**: Hand bones (palm) **Phalanges**: Fingers and thumb
Facial (the major bones) **Mandible**: Lower jaw **Maxilla**: Upper jaw **Ethmoid**: Between nasal cavity and orbits **Sphenoid**: Supports nasal cavity **Zygomatic**: Arch of cheek (high portion)	**Lower Extremities** **Femur (thighbone)**: **largest, longest, strongest bone** **Greater trochanter**: Knob, top of femur **Patella**: Kneecap **Tibia (shinbone)**: Largest lower leg bone **Fibula**: Lower leg bone, lateral side of leg **Tarsals**: Ankle bones, the **calcaneus** (heel bone) is the largest one **Metatarsals**: Foot bones **Phalanges**: Toe bones
Smallest bones of the body: Malleus, incus, stapes (in the ear)	**Scapula (shoulder blade)**: Upper back bone **Clavicle (collarbone)**: Anterior shoulder bone
Column (spine): 26 Bones Cervical: C1–7, curve inward; first, **atlas**: (up-down); second, **axis** (rotation) Thoracic: T1–12, curve outward Lumbar: L1–5, curve inward Sacral: Five fused vertebrae, curve out Coccyx: Four fused vertebrae	**Pelvic girdle**: Basin-shaped **Ilium**: Winged-shaped portion **Ischium**: Inferior portion of hip; sit support **Pubis**: Anterior union of hip bones, **sacrum, coccyx**, and ligaments

Axial Skeleton: The Major Bones	Appendicular Skeleton
Thorax (Ribcage) **Sternum:** Breastbone **(mediastinum)** Xiphoid process: small, flat, bladelike bone tip at bottom of breastbone **Ribs:** 12 Pair	

Your Notes

Diagnostic Testing and Procedures

Arthrocentesis: Puncture to remove fluid for pressure pain relief or analysis.

Arthroscopy: Joint viewing and surgical access.

Laminectomy and spinal fusion: Stabilizes vertebrae by removing part of it.

Traction and reduction: Realigning the bones.

X-ray: Picture of bones for breaks, density.

Common Diseases and Conditions

Carpal tunnel syndrome: Pressure on wrist median nerve

Cleft palate: Congenital deformity

Fractures:

- **Greenstick**: Incomplete break in bone.
- **Simple**: Complete break, does not go through skin.
- **Compound**: Complete break, and also goes through skin.
- **Impacted**: Broken ends are forced into on another.
- **Spiral**: Twisted break of bone.
- **Comminuted**: Several fragments of crushed bone.

Gout: Pain usually affecting great toe area from uric acid buildup.

Kyphosis: Hunchback; outward curve.

Lordosis: Swayback; inward curve.

Osteoarthritis: Inflammation of the joints.

Osteomalacia: Softening of the bone.

Osteoporosis: Bone mass reduction.

Phantom pain: Sensations in an absent amputated limb.

Rheumatoid arthritis: Autoimmune, painful joint swelling resulting in deformities.

Rickets: Lack of vitamin D.

Scoliosis: Lateral, sideward curve.

Spina bifida: Exposed spinal column.

Spondylosis: Inflammation of one or more vertebrae.

Sprain: Tearing of ligaments.

Word Roots	
Root	**Meaning**
cost	Rib
arthr	Joint
ankyl	Crooked, stiff, bent
chondr	Cartilage
kinesi	Movement, motion
lamin	Lamina (thin, flat plate or layer)

Your Notes

Muscular System

Functions	Cells, Tissues, Organs
1. Movement through cellular chemical reactions: muscle contracts—shortens and pulls a bone 2. Maintains posture and alignment 3. Protects bones and internal organs 4. Generates heat	1. Muscles **Smooth**: Involuntary, walls of hollow organs, contractions cause movement **(peristalsis)** **Skeletal (striated)**: Voluntary, attached to bones **Cardiac**: Involuntary, walls of heart, rhythmic cell pulse 2. Tendons: Connective, attach muscle to periosteum of bone 3. Ligaments: Attach bone to bone (anterior cruciate of knee)

Additional Information

Aponeurosis: Broad sheet attaching muscle to muscle or muscles to bones.

Synapses: Junction transmitting messages from nerves to stimulate muscles to act.

Organization: Over 600 Muscles

See diagram for more.

Muscle	Location
Achilles tendon	**Very strong;** attaches gastrocnemius and soleus muscles of lower leg to calcaneus
Biceps	Upper arm bender or flexor
Deltoid	Upper shoulder and arm muscle (site for adult injections)
Gluteus medius	Buttocks, upper outer quadrant (injections at dorso-gluteal or ventrogluteal site)
Masseter	Closes mouth and principal muscle in mastication
Pectoralis major	Chest muscle
Triceps	Upper arm straightener or extensor
Vastus lateralis	Upper outer thigh (common site for infant injections)

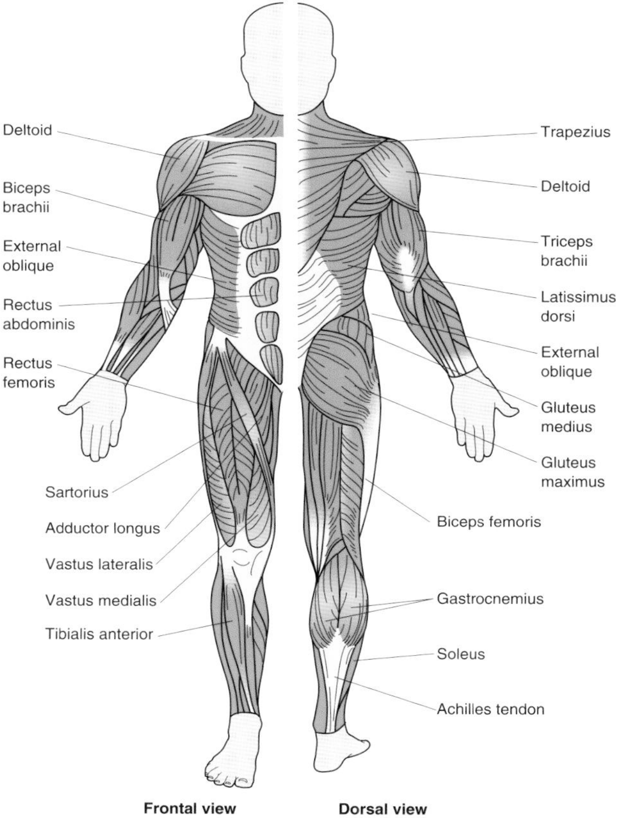

Deltoid
Biceps brachii
External oblique
Rectus abdominis
Rectus femoris
Sartorius
Adductor longus
Vastus lateralis
Vastus medialis
Tibialis anterior

Trapezius
Deltoid
Triceps brachii
Latissimus dorsi
External oblique
Gluteus medius
Gluteus maximus
Biceps femoris
Gastrocnemius
Soleus
Achilles tendon

Frontal view **Dorsal view**

Diagnostic Testing and Procedures

Goniometry: Examining for measurements of joint movement and angles.
Manipulation: Examination; using ROM (range of motion) procedure; using PT (physical therapy).
X-ray: Examination through pictures of muscles.

Common Diseases and Conditions

Atrophy: Muscle wasting due to lack of usage.
Bursitis: Inflammation of bursa (fluid-filled sac that reduces friction as joints move).
Epicondylitis: Inflammation of forearm tendon (tennis elbow).
Muscular dystrophy: Disease of wasting of skeletal muscles.
Myasthenia gravis: Neuromuscular disease, poor transmission from nerves to muscle fibers.
Polymyalgia rheumatica: Muscle pain and stiffness.
Sprain: Overstretching a ligament.
Strain: Overstretching a tendon.
Tendonitis: Inflammation of tendons.

Word Roots

Root	Meaning
aponeur	Aponeurosis
burs	Bursa (cavity)
ten, tend, tendin	Tendon
my, myos	Muscle

Your Notes

Cardiovascular System

Functions	Cells, Tissues, Organs
1. Transports nutrients and oxygen to tissues 2. Transports waste to organs for removal 3. Assists in regulating body temperature 4. Blood cells assist immune system (WBCs) 5. Assist in maintaining proper pH (O_2 and CO_2)	1. Heart 2. Blood: 6 L; 45% are elements in plasma 3. Blood vessels

Organization

Heart

- In pericardium (fluid-filled sac); outer membrane, parietal pericardium; inner membrane, visceral pericardium.
- Four chambers: two upper **atria** (singular, atrium); two lower **ventricles**—left ventricle is larger and thicker.
- **Septum**: Vertically divides heart in half.
- **Mitral (bicuspid) valve**: On left side.
- **Tricuspid valve**: On right side.

Arteries

- Pulsate to transport blood away from heart and have thickest vessel walls.
- Rich with O_2 saturation—except pulmonary artery; exits right side of heart and leads to lungs.

Coronary: Supplying blood for heart muscle function.
Aorta: Largest in the body, carries blood surging from left ventricle of heart.
Carotid: Side of neck, common pulse site.

Brachial: Inside of elbow, used for BP.
Radial: Thumb side of wrist, pulse site.
Femoral: Inner upper thigh, pulse site.

Arterioles

Downsized arteries, connect to capillaries.

Veins

- Contain many valves to prevent blood backflow and transport blood to heart.
- Have poor O_2 saturation, except pulmonary vein; enters left side of heart with O_2-rich blood from lungs.

Vena cava: Drains upper (superior vena cava) and lower (inferior vena cava) parts of body.
Median cephalic vein: Usual venipuncture site (inside bend of elbow).

Venules

Downsized veins, smaller and thinner, connect to capillaries.

Capillaries

- One cell layer thick.
- Allow for exchange of nutrients and waste products throughout body.

Blood

- Most formed in red bone marrow.
- Plasma: Liquid portion of blood suspending cells.

Red blood cells (RBCs): Biconcave, contain hgb, live 120 days, carry O_2 and CO_2, avg. count 5,000,000/mm^3.
Platelets: Thrombocytes, cell fragments; help blood clot, avg. count 200,000/mm^3.
White blood cells (WBCs): Fight infection, avg. count 5,000 to 10,000/mm^3.

- **Five types**
  - **Agranulocytes** (formed in lymphatic system)
    - Lymphocytes, monocytes.
  - **Granulocytes** (formed in red bone marrow)
    - Neutrophils (most numerous), basophils, eosinophils.

Diagnostic Testing and Procedures

Arteriogram: X-ray of arteries.
EKG (ECG): Printed tracing of cardiac rhythm.
Stress test: Measurement of heart activity during physical activity.

Common Diseases and Conditions

Anemia: Abnormally ↓ hemoglobin or RBCs
Angina pectoris: ↓ O_2 to heart, causes severe chest pain; due to stress or activity.
Aneurysm: Out-pouching of weakened blood vessel wall; due to trauma or genetic cause.
Arteriosclerosis: Hardening of arteries.
Atherosclerosis: Fatty plaque buildup in coronary arteries, ↓ blood flow to heart muscle.
Bradycardia: Slow cardiac rhythm, ↓ 60 beats per minute.
Congestive heart failure (CHF): Pulmonary edema resulting from ↓ pumping performance of heart.
Claudication: Circulation problem; calf pain upon walking, subsides at rest.
Heart block: Interruption of heart's electrical conduction from SA node to AV node.
Hemophilia: Inability to clot blood.
Hypertension: High BP, ↑ 140/90.
Ischemia: Temporary ↓ of blood flow to an organ or tissue.
Murmur: Blood leaking back through a narrowed or deformed valve.
MI (myocardial infarction): Heart attack, results in some cardiac muscle necrosis.
Rheumatic heart disease: Damaged coronary valves resulting from streptococcal upper respiratory infection (URI)
Tachycardia: Rapid cardiac rhythm, ↑ 100 beats per minute.

Word Roots	
Root	**Meaning**
angi	Vessel
ather	Yellowish, fatty plaque
cardi, coron	Heart
isch	Deficiency, blockage
phleb, ven	Vein
sphygm	Pulse
ech	Sound

Your Notes

Lymphatic and Immune System

Functions	Cells, Tissues, Organs
1. Disease defense: active/passive immunity 2. Stores red blood cells 3. Returns excess interstitial fluid to blood 4. Produces lymphocytes 5. Transports lipids	1. Lymph 2. Lymphocytes 3. Lymph nodes 4. Lymphatic vessels 5. Spleen 6. Tonsils: three pair—palatine, pharyngeal, lingual 7. Thymus

Immunity

Active	Passive
Natural: Produced by body's production of antibodies after exposure to disease-causing organism.	**Natural**: Maternal antibodies produced outside body and passed on while breast feeding or in the uterus.
Artificial: Acquired from immunizations composed of dead or weakened organisms, inactivated toxins or recombinant DNA. Body produces antibodies to become immune.	**Artificial**: Acquired from immunizations composed of antibodies or globulins to readily fight specific disease-causing organisms, if exposed.

Organization

Lymph: Tissue Fluid

- Formed from plasma; composed of water, electrolytes, metabolizing cell waste, protein.

Lymphocytes: WBCs

Defense against pathogens.

T cells mature in thymus, reside in lymph tissue and blood.
T cells attack through cell-to-cell contact **(cell-mediated immunity) phagocytosis.**
B cells mature in bone marrow and reside in lymph tissue and blood.
B cells indirectly attack by secreting **antibodies (antibody-mediated immunity).**

Lymph Nodes

- Pea-shaped clusters of lymph tissue, filter microorganisms from lymph as it flows.
- Through lymph vessels; large cluster locations include **axillary lymph nodes; inguinal lymph nodes; cervical lymph nodes.**

Lymphatic Vessels

- Extensive network, every body organ has them.
- Lymph from right arm and right side of head drain into **right lymphatic duct.**
- Lymph from rest of body drains into **thoracic duct.**

Spleen: Largest Lymphoid Organ

- Filters blood, a blood reservoir.
- Destroys old RBCs, and has role in erythropoiesis.

Tonsils: Three Pairs

- **Palatine**: Mostly removed in tonsillectomy.
- **Pharyngeal**: Also called adenoids.
- **Lingual**: Located in back of tongue.

Thymus

- Mostly active during early life.
- Produces thymosin for maturation and function of T-cell lymphocytes.

Diagnostic Testing and Procedures

Allergy testing: Methods include scratch test, patch test, intradermal test, radioallergosorbent test (RAST).

Complete blood count (CBC): Includes hemoglobin, hematocrit, RBC and WBC count.

EIA (enzyme immunoassay): First test for HIV, usually on venous blood.

Liver function: Measure coagulation factors, prothrombin and fibrinogen.

WBC differential: Classification of cells; check for immunity, infection, allergies.

Western blot: Confirmatory test for HIV.

Common Diseases and Conditions

Allergic response disorder: Hypersensitivities—contact dermatitis, anaphylaxis.

Autoimmune disorder: Immune system produces antibodies against its own cells.

Immunodeficiency disease: Incompetent or deficient immune system.

- **SCID**: Congenital—children succumb to minor infections.
- **AIDS**: Viral-induced—onset as HIV has ↑ T-cell count than AIDS.

Lymphoma: Benign or malignant tumor.

- **Hodgkin's disease**: Malignant with enlarged spleen, generally in young men.
- **Non-Hodgkin's lymphoma**: Malignant throughout lymph tissues, generally in older adults.

Mononucleosis (mono): Caused by Epstein-Barr virus, enlarged spleen and lymph tissue.

Splenomegaly: Enlarged spleen, associated with infectious disease.

Word Roots

Root	Meaning
lymph	Lymph
spleen	Spleen
thym	Thymus

Your Notes

Digestive System

Functions	Cells, Tissues, Organs
1. Digestion 2. Absorption 3. Elimination	1. Mouth 2. Pharynx 3. Esophagus 4. Stomach 5. Small intestines and large intestines 6. Liver 7. Gallbladder 8. Pancreas

Organization

Mouth: Where digestion starts.

- **Mastication** mixes food with saliva forming a **bolus.**
- Tongue has **frenulum linguae**: tissue that anchors tongue to mouth floor.

Pharynx: Passes bolus to esophagus.

Esophagus: Tube between pharynx and stomach.

- **Epiglottis**: Covers larynx (windpipe) when swallowing, bolus then enters esophagus.

Stomach: Composed of **rugae cells.**

- Mixes food with gastric acids to form **chyme.**

Small intestines: Longest portion of intestines; most nutrients absorbed here.

Peristalsis: Rhythmic movement of chyme through small and large intestines.

Duodenum: First section, bile from gallbladder and pancreatic juices enter.

Jejunum: Second part, middle portion.

Ileum: Last part of small intestine.

Large intestines: Where elimination occurs.

- Normal flora here produce vitamin K.

Cecum: Blind pouch at beginning, lower portion is **appendix** .

- **McBurney's point**: Site of tenderness associated with appendicitis.

Colon: Three parts:

- **Ascending:** R side of abdomen, vertical.
- **Transverse**: Middle portion, horizontal.
- **Descending:** L side of abdomen, vertical.

Sigmoid: S-shaped, connects colon to rectum.
Rectum: Connects sigmoid to anus.
Anus: Final portion, where feces are excreted.

Accessory Organs of Digestion

Liver: Produces bile, cholesterol; stores glycogen, vitamins B_{12}, A, D, E, K; detoxifies blood; aids metabolism.
Gallbladder: Stores and secretes bile to aid in digestion and fats emulsion.
Pancreas: An **endocrine gland**—secretes insulin into bloodstream; an **exocrine organ**—produces pancreatic juices for digestion.

Diagnostic Testing and Procedures

Cholecystography: X-ray of gallbladder.
Colonoscopy, sigmoidoscopy, proctoscopy: Viewing parts of large intestine.
Lower GI: Barium enema used to x-ray lower GI tract.
Upper GI: Barium swallow used to x-ray upper GI tract.

Common Diseases and Conditions

Anorexia: No appetite, aversion to food.
Botulism: Food poisoning, usual cause is *Clostridium botulinum* bacteria.
Cholelithiasis: Gallstones; painful, nausea, vomiting, mild jaundice.
Cirrhosis: End-stage liver disease, chronic liver cell destruction.
Colitis: Inflammation of colon.
Crohn's disease: Inflammatory bowel disease, usually ileum.
Diverticula: Abnormal pouching (pocketing) of organ walls; usually colon.

Hemorrhoids: Dilated, inflamed veins of rectum and anus.
Hepatitis: Inflammation of liver; eight types—A, B, C, D, E, F, G, H.
Hernia: Protrusion of an organ through the wall of containing cavity.
IBS (irritable bowel syndrome): Inflammation of colon, may be related to food or stress.
Ulcers: Lesions of mucous membrane lining of an organ.

Additional Information

Construction by adhesions: Abnormal growing together of two surfaces, normally separated.
Flatus: Gas in digestive tract or expelled through anus.
Gavage: Process of feeding a person through a nasogastric tube.
Ascites: Abnormal collection of fluid in the peritoneal cavity.
Intussusception: Telescoping/sliding of one part of intestine into another.
Volvulus: Twisting or kinking of the intestine.

Word Roots

Root	Meaning
an	Anus
cec	Cecum
cheil	Lip
chol	Gall, bile
cholangi	Bile duct
choledoch	Common bile duct
enter	Intestines, usually small
gastr	Stomach
gingiv	Gum
gloss, lingu	Tongue
hepat	Liver
lapar, celi	Abdomen; abdominal cavity
sial	Saliva
stomat, or	Mouth

Your Notes

Integumentary System

Functions	Cells, Tissues, Organs
1. Controls body temperature 2. First line of defense from infection 3. Assists in preventing dehydration	1. Skin: epidermis, dermis, subcutaneous 2. Glands: sweat, ceruminous, sebaceous **Accessory Components** 3. Hair 4. Nails

Organization

Skin

Largest organ, covers all of body.

Epidermis: Outermost, skin surface; single cell layers (strata)

- Holds **melanin:** pigment that gives skin its color.
- Receptor for touch.
- Prevents water loss, by way of **keratin.**

Dermis: "True skin," middle layer; contains blood vessels, nerves and nerve endings, glands.

Subcutaneous: Innermost, fatty layer. contains adipose tissue, elastic fibers that adhere dermis to muscle surfaces, provides body with fuel, retains heat, cushion for inner tissues.

Glands: Located in Dermis Layer

Sweat glands: Produce and secrete sweat to assist in body temperature regulation and rid body of waste.

Sebaceous glands: Near hair follicles; secrete oily **sebum** to lubricate skin and hair.

Ceruminous: In ear; secrete **cerumen** (earwax) for protection.

Hair

- Composed mostly of **keratin** tissue.
- Found on most of body.
- Center of hair shaft called the **medulla**.

Nails

- Composed of hardened **keratin (horny layer)**; found on tips of fingers and toes.

Diagnostic Testing and Procedures

Diascope: Examination of skin lesions using flat glass plate held against skin.

"Rule of Nines": Used to determine percentage of body that has been burned.

Surgical excision and biopsy: Done for lesions and moles to detect cancer cells.

Sweat chloride test: Used to detect cystic fibrosis, checks salt content of sweat.

Wood's light: Fluorescent light used to diagnose particular skin conditions.

Common Diseases and Conditions

Acne: Inflammation of sebaceous glands.

Albinism: Absence of melanin (pigment) in skin, hair, eyes.

Alopecia: Absence of hair to entire body or area.

Burns

- First degree: Superficial, only epidermis, little edema; rug burn.
- Second degree: Partial thickness; epidermis, part of dermis, blistering and edema.
- Third degree: Full thickness; pale or charred appearance with edema.

Carcinoma (skin cancer)

- Basal cell: Basal cell layer, slow spreading, usual to fair skin.
- Squamous cell: Squamous cell layer, metastasizes ↑ than basal.
- Malignant melanoma: Usually a mole, metastasizes quickly.

Dermatitis: Inflammation of skin causing itching and redness.
Diaphoresis: Excessive sweating.
Eczema: Dry leather patches, vesicles; causes itching.
Furuncle: Boil.
Herpes virus

- Simplex: Cold sore or fever blister.
- Zoster (shingles): Painful vesicles on nerve endings; causes chicken pox.

Impetigo: Contagious bacterial skin infection, caused by streptococcus or staphylococcus.
Keloid: Abnormal scar, raised.
Macule: Flat skin lesion; white, brown, or red (freckle).
Nevus: Mole; raised congenital spot on skin surface.
Papule: Pimple.
Pediculosis: Infestation by lice; usually on head.
Psoriasis: Inflammation of skin; scaly red raised patches on skin surface; causes itching.
Scabies: Infection caused by mite burrowing under skin; causes itching.
Scleroderma: Causes thickened, rigid skin.
Tinea: Fungal skin infection (e.g., ringworm, athlete's foot).
Tinea capitis: "Cradle cap."
Urticaria: Hives or raised wheals caused by allergic reaction or stress.
Vesicle: Raised blister-like sac on skin.

Word Roots

Root	Meaning
cutaine, derm, dermat	Skin
hidr	Sweat
kerat	Horny tissue, hard
onych, ungu	Nail
trich	Hair
crypt	Hidden
heter	Other
myc	Fungus
pachy	Thick
rhytid	Wrinkles
xer	Dry

Your Notes

Respiratory System

Functions	Cells, Tissues, Organs	
	Upper Tract	**Lower Tract**
1. Inhalation: inhaling nutrients to body (e.g., O_2) 2. Exhalation: exhaling body waste products (CO_2) 3. Diffusion: supplying and removing gases to blood	1. Nose 2. Sinuses 3. Mouth 4. Pharynx 5. Epiglottis 6. Larynx	1. Trachea 2. Bronchi 3. Alveoli 4. Lungs 5. Pleura 6. Thorax 7. Diaphragm

Organization

Upper Respiratory Tract: Passageway from Outside Body to Lungs	Lower Respiratory Tract
Nose • Lined with cilia and hair to clean air • Warm, clean, and moisturize air	**Trachea** • Tube in front of neck with C-shaped rings
Sinuses: Air Spaces in Bones of Face • Lined with ciliated mucous membrane • Warm, clean, and moisturize air	**Bronchi** • Two stem off trachea, one to each lung • Smaller branches called bronchioles
Mouth • When extra air is needed • No moisturizing capacity of nose	**Alveoli** • Air sacs, bronchiole ends; one cell thick • Where exchange of gases occurs

Upper Respiratory Tract: Passageway from Outside Body to Lungs	Lower Respiratory Tract
Pharynx—throat; passageway for air and food from mouth to **hyoid** bone	**Lungs—main organ;** in thoracic cavity • L one has two lobes, R one has three lobes
Epiglottis—cartilage flap, functions as a valve; moves to cover trachea as you swallow	**Pleura** • Serous membrane lining lungs; has surfactant to ↓ surface tension
Larynx—"voice box," just below epiglottis • Cartilage and muscle • A backup for epiglottis, closes when swallowing • Contains vocal cords to produce voice	**Thorax** • Cavity containing lungs **Diaphragm** • Domed muscle, separates thoracic cavity and abdominal cavity • On inhalation; diaphragm contracts (creating room for inflation of lungs) • On exhalation; diaphragm relaxes (assists lung compression)

Additional Information

Expiratory reserve volume: Extra air forcibly exhaled after normal exhalation.

External respiration: Exchange of O_2 and CO_2 in lungs and blood capillaries.

Functional residual volume: Amount of air left in lungs after normal expiration.

Inspiratory capacity (inspiratory reserve volume): Maximum amount of air inspired after normal expiration; breath in/out normally, then forcibly inhale at end of tidal volume.

Internal respiration: Exchange of O_2 and CO_2 between capillaries and tissue cells.

Rales (rhonchi): Increased secretions in bronchi causing crackling breath sounds.

Residual volume: Volume of air left in lungs after forced expiration.

Tidal volume: Volume of air inspired and expired during a normal respiration.

Total lung capacity: Total volume of air that can be in lungs at one time.

Vital capacity: Maximum amount of air expired after maximum inspiration; not forced.

Wheeze: Squeaking, whistling breath sounds in asthma; narrowed tracheobronchial airways.

Diagnostic Testing and Procedures

Bronchoscopy: Viewing tissues of lungs.

Chest x-ray: Radiological picture of lungs.

Pulmonary function tests: Spirometry used to measure various lung capacities.

Common Diseases and Conditions

Asthma: Wheezing or severe dyspnea due to narrowed airways, usually allergy-related.

Atelectasis: Absence of air in lung(s) and alveoli, cause structures to collapse.

Bronchitis: Inflammation of bronchi.

Chronic obstructive: Usually progressive; obstructs air exchange in bronchi, alveoli and lungs.

Croup: Viral; usually in infants, causes pronounced barking cough.

Cystic fibrosis: Genetic; abnormally thick mucus secretions result in impaired breathing.

Emphysema: Form of COPD, loss of alveoli elasticity, causes difficult respiration.

Legionnaires' disease: Form of pneumonia; caused by *Legionella pneumophila* bacteria.

Pertussis (whooping cough): Bacterial infection (vaccine for it); may be fatal to infants.

Pharyngitis: Inflammation of the pharynx, resulting in a sore throat.

Pleurisy: Inflammation of pleura, breathing may be painful.
Pneumonia: Infection of lung tissue, air has difficulty reaching alveoli.
Pneumothorax: Air in pleural cavity causing partial or complete collapse of lungs.
Pulmonary edema: Fluid accumulation in lungs, associated with CHF.
Rhinitis: Sneezing, watery eyes, nasal drip.
Tuberculosis (TB): Bacterial infection causing nodules in lungs.

Word Roots

Root	Meaning
lob	Lobe
nas, rhin	Nose
pneum, pneumat, pneumon	Lung, air
pulmon	Lung
muc	Mucus
ox	Oxygen
py	Pus
spir	Breathe, breathing

Your Notes

Nervous System

Functions	Cells, Tissues, Organs
1. Controls and integrates body activities 2. Adjusts body functions for homeostasis 3. Initiates thoughts and emotions 4. Generates sensations 5. Receptors for smell, taste, sound, vision	**Central Nervous System (CNS)** 1. Brain 2. Spinal cord **Peripheral Nervous System (PNS)** 1. Spinal nerves and ganglia 2. Cranial nerves and ganglia

Additional Information

Afferent system: Sends info from receptors to CNS.

Autonomic system: Sends info from CNS to smooth muscle, cardiac muscle and glands.

Blood-brain barrier: Regulates what materials in bloodstream can enter brain.

Efferent system: Sends info from CNS to muscles and glands.

Parasympathetic nervous system: Responsible for conservation/ restoration of energy and elimination of waste.

Somatic system: Sends info from CNS to skeletal muscles.

Sympathetic nervous system: Responsible for automatic reactions to stress; "Flight or Fight Syndrome."

Organization

Neuron: Nerve Cell

Cell body: Protected in brain, spinal cord, or ganglion

Dendrite: Have receptors to pick up stimuli and carry to cell body

Axon: Carry impulses to other neurons or body tissues

Myelin (lipid and protein) sheath: Covers axon

- Made from **Schwann cells**; gaps called **"nodes of Ranvier," "white matter"** nerve cells.
- CNS neurons do not have this, cannot repair, they are **"gray matter"** cells.

Synapse: Gap between neurons and/or muscle tissue.

- A released neurotransmitter chemical assists impulse transmission.

Sensory neurons: Transmit impulses from rest of body to CNS.
Motor neurons: Transmit impulses from CNS to muscles and glands.
Interneurons: Bridge between sensory and motor neurons; all are located in CNS.

Brain

Encephalon, 3 lbs.

- Protected by skull, meninges, CSF (cerebrospinal fluid).
- Outer surface—gray matter: thinking, reasoning.
- Inside-white matter: bundles of nerve fibers carry info to and from cortex.

Main Sections

Cerebral hemispheres (left, right cerebrum)

- Largest part.
- Sensory, motor, intellect; covered with gray matter called cerebral cortex.
- Shallow folds: **sulci;** L side for logic, complex math, language; R side for creativity, music and art appreciation.

Diencephalon: Contains thalamus, hypothalamus, pineal gland.

- Link between where decisions made and body carries out.

Cerebellum: Little brain.

- Maintains muscle tone, balance, posture, fine motor movement.

Hindbrain (brainstem)—three parts:

- **Medulla oblongata:** Lowest part; channels communication between spinal cord and brain.
- **Pons (bridge):** Helps regulate breathing.
- **Midbrain:** Nerve tissue; connects pons to ↓ part of cerebrum; vision and hearing reflexes.

Cranial Nerves

I. **Olfactory**: Sense of smell
II. **Optic**: Vision
III. **Oculomotor**: Movement of eyeball, eyelid, regulation of pupil size
IV. **Trochlear**: Movement of eyeball
V. **Trigeminal**: Sensation in head and face, chewing
VI. **Abducens:** Eye movement
VII. **Facial**: Taste, facial expressions, secretions of tears and saliva
VIII. **Acoustic**: Hearing, balance
IX. **Glossopharyngeal**: Taste, swallowing, secretion of saliva
X. **Vagus**: Sensation in larynx, trachea, heart, stomach, and other organs; organ movement
XI. **Spinal accessory**: Movement of shoulders and head
XII. **Hypoglossal**: Tongue movement

Hemisphere Brain Lobes

Frontal: Controls speech and voluntary muscle movement.
Parietal: Sensory area from skin; depth perception, size, shape.
Temporal: Sound and smell interpretation; personality, behavior, emotion, memory.
Occipital: Interprets sight.

Spinal Cord

Gray and white matter.

- Begins at base of brain (**medulla oblongata**) and extends to second lumbar vertebra in adults.
- Protected by **bone**: skull and vertebrae.

Meninges (membranes): dura mater (outermost layer); arachnoid (lacy spiderweb); pia mater (innermost layer).
CSF: In subarachnoid space, between arachnoid and pia mater.

- Thirty-one pairs of spinal nerves, named for the vertebrae they correspond to.

Diagnostic Testing and Procedures

Angiography: Use contrast medium to view blood vessels of brain.
CAT scan (computed axial tomography): Pictures of brain layers to clearly see components.
EEG (electroencephalogram): Measures electrical activity of brain.
Lumbar puncture: Extraction of CSF below L3 or L4 for examination.
MRI (magnetic resonance imaging): Brain pictures using magnetic waves of soft tissue.
Myelogram: Radio-opaque medium to view interior of spinal cord.
Patellar, Babinski, Achilles, and corneal reflexes: Reflex tests for motor neuron function.
X-rays (skull and spine): To diagnose injuries, tumors, spondylitis of vertebrae.

Common Diseases and Conditions

Alzheimer's disease: Degenerative; dementia-like; ↓ of intellect, memory, physical abilities.
Bell's palsy: Bacterial infection, causes one-sided facial paralysis; affects cranial nerve VII.
Carpal tunnel syndrome: Fluid puts pressure on nerves in carpal area; numbness, pain.
Cerebral palsy: Brain damage in utero or birth; mental retardation, seizures, spastic moves.
CVA (cerebrovascular accident; stroke): Brain circulation block or vessel rupture; location affects body function.
Epilepsy: Malfunction of electrical activity of brain; causes periodic seizures.
Hydrocephalus: Excessive fluid in brain causing elevated pressure and tissue death.
Meningitis: Viral or bacterial infection of meninges covering brain.
Multiple sclerosis: Progressive; gaps in myelin sheath; weakness, tremors, vision problems.
Parkinson's disease: Progressive; ↓ supply of dopamine; tremors, involuntary movement.
Sciatica: Inflammation of sciatic nerve.

TIA (transient ischemic attack): Minor, temporary symptoms, warning of possible upcoming stroke.

Types of Seizures

Petit mal: Usually occurs in childhood; mental shutdown ("go blank") for up to 30 seconds; patient doesn't know what is happening and after episode doesn't know it occurred.

Grand mal: Occurs at any age; patient falls down unconscious, goes rigid, twitches or jerks rhythmically; slowly regains consciousness; usually followed by deep sleep or confusion; may be preceded by an "aura" or warning.

Focal seizure: Uncontrollable twitching; begins on one part of body (e.g., thumb) then spreads to surrounding structures and eventually full body; patient is conscious during seizure.

Temporal lobe seizure: After brief aura, or warning, the patient suddenly acts out of character for a few minutes, an unconscious chewing motion may occur during seizure.

Word Roots

Root	Meaning
cerebell	Cerebellum (hindbrain)
cerebr	Cerebrum
dur	Hard (dura mater)
encephal	Brain
radic, radicul, rhiz	Nerve root
esthesi	Sensation, sensitivity, feeling
phas	Speech
poli	Gray matter
psych, ment, phren	Mind

Your Notes

Special Senses

Gustatory (Taste), Olfactory (SMELL), Vision, and Hearing	
Functions	**Gustatory Components**
1. Taste	1. Papillae
	2. Soft palate
	Olfactory Components
2. Smell	1. Mucous lining (nasal epithelium)
3. Vision	**Vision Components**
	1. Eyelids, Eyelashes, Eyebrows, Tears
	2. Lacrimal glands
	3. Outer layer
	4. Second layer
	5. Third layer
	6. Interior
	Hearing Components
4. Hearing	1. Outer ear
5. Sense of balance or position	2. Middle ear
	3. Inner ear

Organization

Gustatory Components

Receptors for taste mostly on tongue and soft palate.

Papillae: Raised areas on tongue; detect only four "tastes"—sweet, salt, sour, bitter.

Olfactory Components

Smell receptors in mucous lining of ↑ part of nose.

Vision Components

Receptors for vision are in retina.

Eyelids, Eyelashes, Eyebrows, Tears: Protective structures for eye, clean and moisturize eye.

Lacrimal glands: On outside upper edge of each eye; secrete tears.

Outer layer of eye

- **Sclera**: White of eye.
- **Cornea**: "Window"; transparent front of eye; allows light to enter eye.

Second layer of eye

- **Iris:** "Rainbow," beneath cornea and in front of lens; has opening in center known as **pupil**.

Third layer of eye

- **Retina**: Lines interior of eyeball; **rods** (seeing gray tones) and **cones** (light and color) found at back of interior.

Interior of Eye

- **Lens:** Below cornea and iris; enables eye to focus (process called **accommodation).**
- **Vitreous humor**: Behind lens; jelly-like substance; maintains shape of eye and support retina.

Hearing Components

Outer ear

- **Pinna (auricle)**: Skin, cartilage outside ear.

Eardrum: External auditory, then membrane; vibrates as sound waves hit it.

Middle ear: connected to nasopharynx by **eustachian tube.**

- **Malleus, incus, stapes (ossicles)**: Move and pass vibrations from middle to inner ear.

Inner ear (labyrinth)

- **Vestibule**: Small chamber, concerned with balance.
- **Semicircular canals:** Concerned with balance.
- **Cochlea:** Stapes communicates to cochlea; spiral-shape; contains fluid sacs and tubes.

Additional Information

Blind spot (optic disc): No rods and cones; where optic nerve leaves eyeball.

Diagnostic Testing and Procedures

Audiometry: Emitting measured sounds to evaluate hearing.
Electrocochleography: Measure electrical activity in cochlea.
Refraction: Checking for visual correction or glasses.
Tonometry: Intraocular pressure testing (a check for glaucoma).
Visual acuity: Snellen chart, Ishihara method—distance and near vision testing, color vision test.

Common Diseases and Conditions

Amblyopia: Eye not used is "lazy eye," becomes progressively weaker.
Astigmatism: Distortion caused by uneven curvature of cornea.
Cataract: Cloudiness (opacity) of eye lens; aging degeneration.
Color blindness: At birth, mostly males, absence or deficiency of one type of cone.
Conjunctivitis (pink eye): Conjunctiva inflammation, eye white turns red/pink; contagious.
Exophthalmia: Bulging (protrusion) of eyes out of orbits; usual cause is hyperthyroidism.
Glaucoma: ↑ Pressure on optic nerve; can cause blindness, O_2 can't reach rods and cones.
Hypermetropia: Farsightedness, eye is too short from front to back.
Iritis: Inflamed iris tissue; cells from area flake off, can interfere with vision.
Macular degeneration: ↑ Growth of blood vessels in retina; progressive, causes blindness.
Ménière's disease: ↑ Fluid in semicircular canals; symptoms are dizziness, hearing loss, ringing in ears.
Myopia: Nearsightedness, eye is too long from cornea to retina.
Night blindness: Lack of vitamin A.
Otitis externa: Swimmer's ear.
Otitis media: Middle ear infection, starts at throat, goes up Eustachian tube, common in infants.
Otosclerosis: Partial deafness due to abnormal bone growth, stapes becomes immobilized.
Presbyopia: Hardening, loss of flexibility in eye lens; happens with age.
Strabismus: "Cross-eyed," poor alignment of eye muscles.

Stye: Eyelash follicle infection.
Vertigo: Dizziness.

Word Roots

Root	Meaning
blephar	Eyelid
cor, core, pupil	Pupil
corne, kerat	Cornea
dacry, lacrim	Tear, tear duct
ocul, ophthalm	Eye
opt	Vision
cry	Cold
phot	Light
ton	Tension, pressure
acou, audi	Hearing
aur, ot	Ear
miring	Tympanic membrane (eardrum)
tympan	Eardrum, middle ear

Your Notes

Endocrine System

Functions	Cells, Tissues, Organs
1. Works with nervous system; provides hormone needs 2. Control rates of certain chemical reactions 3. Helps transport substances through membranes 4. Helps regulate water and electrolyte balance 5. Role in growth, development, and reproductive processes	1. Hypothalamus gland 2. Pituitary gland (under brain) 3. Pineal gland (center of brain) 4. Thyroid gland (below larynx) 5. Parathyroid glands (thyroid lobes) 6. Adrenal glands (kidney tops) 7. Pancreas (in duodenum curve) 8. Gonads (sex glands)

Additional Information

Acidosis: Abnormal accumulation of acid products of metabolism; seen frequently in uncontrolled diabetes mellitus.

Hypothalamus: Master of the "master gland," secretions control hormones secreted by pituitary.

Metabolism: Sum total of all chemical processes that take place in a living organism.

Pituitary gland: The "master gland."

Syndrome: Set of symptoms that run (occur) together.

Organization

Hormone	Target	Major Functions
Anterior Pituitary		
GH (growth hormone)	Bone, muscle, soft tissue	Stimulate tissue growth; decreases glucose
Prolactin	Mammary glands (breasts)	Initiates milk production; promotes milk gland production
TSH (thyroid stimulating hormone)	Thyroid gland	Growth, development and thyroid activity as metabolism regulator
ACTH (adrenocorticotropin hormone)	Adrenal glands (cortex)	Maintenance of gland, stimulates secretion of cortisol
FSH (follicle stimulating hormone)	Ovarian follicles; seminiferous tubules in testes	**Women,** stimulates development of ova and ovulation, secretion of estrogen; **men,** stimulates development and function of testes, production of sperm
LH (luteinizing hormone)	Ovaries; testes—cells of Leydig	Development of corpus luteum, progesterone secretion; develops cells to make testosterone, stimulates secretion of testosterone
Posterior Pituitary		
ADH (antidiuretic hormone), vasopressin	Kidneys	Regulates water reabsorption within nephrons, determines urine concentration and volume

Continued

Hormone	Target	Major Functions
Oxytocin	Uterus; breasts	Stimulates birth contractions and causes milk ejection
Thyroid Gland		
T4 (thyroxine)	Tissue cells	Increases metabolic rate
T3 (tri-iodothyronine)	Tissue cells	Increases metabolic rate
Calcitonin	Bone	Inhibits bone ↓, ↓ blood calcium concentration
Parathyroid Glands		
Parathyroid hormone (parathormone)	Intestines, bones	↑ Absorption of calcium into bloodstream; ↑ excretion of phosphates in urine
Adrenal Cortex (Outer)		
Cortisol (ACTH)	All cells except liver cells	↑ Breakdown of proteins into amino acids; breakdown of fats; assists in stress; ↑ blood glucose
Aldosterone	Kidneys	Regulates blood pH; stimulates reabsorption of sodium in nephrons
Androgens	Gonads	Stimulates development of secondary sex characteristics (especially females)
Adrenal Medulla		
Epinephrine (adrenalin)	Smooth and cardiac muscle, blood vessels, liver cells	↑ Heart rate, blood pressure, blood glucose levels

Hormone	Target	Major Functions
Norepinephrine	Smooth, cardiac, and striated muscle	Constricts blood vessels, ↑ BP; reinforces sympathetic nervous system
Pancreas Gland		
Glucagon	Liver cells, fat cells	Promotes release of glucose into blood
Insulin	All cells except brain cells	Promotes use and storage of glucose into cells
Pineal Gland		
Melatonin	Pituitary (LH); gonads	Regulates sexual development, timing of puberty
Thymus Gland		
Thymosin	Immune system	Stimulates T-cell production
Male Gonads (Testes)		
Testosterone	Sperm cells	Stimulates sperm product, and secondary sex characteristics
Female Gonads (Ovaries)		
Estrogen	Breasts, uterus	Stimulates breast growth, uterus and secondary sex characteristics
Progesterone	Uterine lining	Prepares uterus for pregnancy

Diagnostic Testing and Procedures

Bone density x-ray: Using hip bone to see level of calcium ↓.

CAT scan of various glands: Done to seek cause of gland ↑ or ↓ hormone production.

Fasting plasma glucose test: Test normal blood glucose level.

Glucose tolerance test (GTT): Timed; effective rate of glucose absorption into cells.

Thyroid scan, radioimmunoassay (RIA): Rates thyroid activity for metabolic regulation.

24-Hour urine collection: Concentration and levels of glucose, calcium, steroid, K, etc.

Common Diseases and Conditions

Acromegaly: ↑ Growth hormone in adults; usual cause is pituitary gland tumor.

Addison's disease: Bronze skin, hypotension; due to slow destroying of adrenal cortex and ↓ ACTH.

Cretinism: Hypothyroidism in infants and children; abnormally developing brain.

Cushing's syndrome: "Moon face," thin limbs, fat torso; due to adrenal gland tumor and ↑ ACTH.

Diabetes insipidus: ↓ of ADH; polydipsia and polyuria, dehydration, dry skin.

Diabetes mellitus: Caused by insulin ↓ or insulin resistance.

- **Type 1:** Insulin dependent (IDDM), juvenile onset, before age 30—heredity, virus result.
- **Type 2:** Non-insulin dependent (NIDDM), adult onset—obesity, pregnancy.

Goiter: Swollen neck from enlarged thyroid; iodine deficiency, ↓ or ↑ thyroid.

Graves' disease: ↑ Metabolism, exophthalmia, anxiety; thyrotoxicosis due to hyperthyroidism.

Hashimoto's disease: Congenital, autoimmune, hypothyroidism.

Myxedema: Lack of thyroid hormones in adults.

Tetany: Muscle spasms and convulsions; lack of calcium circulating, hypoparathyroidism.

SAD: Seasonal affective disorder, depressive mood disorder; melatonin-related.

Word Roots

Root	Meaning
acr	Extremities, height
calc	Calcium
dips	Thirst
kal	Potassium
toxic	Poison

Your Notes

Urinary System

Functions	Cells, Tissues, Organs
1. Body waste elimination through blood filtration	1. Kidneys (2)
2. Balance of fluids and electrolytes of body	2. Ureters (2)
3. Assistance in detoxification of liver	3. Bladder
4. Regulation of blood chemical makeup	4. Urethra

Organization

Blood Circulation in the Kidney

- Blood enters kidney through renal artery.
- Each minute the heart pumps about one fifth (1,200 mL) of blood supply through kidneys.

Kidneys

Second to the brain in complexity.

- Between 12th thoracic vertebra and third lumbar vertebra, behind abdominal cavity.
- Kidney bean shape: concave side center called **hilus**: renal artery enters here, ureter and renal vein exit here.
- Secrete **erythropoietin,** which acts to stimulate the production of RBCs.

Anatomy of Kidney

Cortex: Outer portion

Medulla: inner portion: Contains about 12 ▲ structures, **pyramids;** each ▲ connects with a **calyx** (duct) and joins a **renal pelvis** (urine reservoir); a **ureter** attached to each renal pelvis.

Nephrons: Kidney functioning unit.

- Approximately 1.25 million per kidney.
- Each is surrounded by blood capillaries.

- Has three functions: filtration, reabsorption, secretion.
- Nephron parts are:
  1. **Glomerulus**: Blood enters nephron here.
  2. **Bowman's capsule**: Blood filtration here.
  3. **Proximal tubule**: Reabsorption begins; concentration/chemical content of urine determined.
  4. **Loop of Henle**: Urine formation continues.
  5. **Distal tubule**: Last area of urine formation.
  6. **Collecting duct**: Urine formation completed; leads to pyramids.

Ureters

- Extend from hilus of kidney to lower surface of bladder.
- Urine is propelled through ureters by **peristalsis** and flows through mucous flap into bladder.

Bladder

- Mucous membrane lining of **rugae** cells (empty bladder will fold); 350–450 mL capacity.
- 150–250 mL of urine enough to stimulate **micturition** (voiding of urine).
- Point where urine exits bladder is **internal sphincter** (involuntary muscle) located at opening where urethra connects to bladder.

Urethra

- About 4 cm long in female and 20 cm long in male.
- Female: Leads directly from bladder to **urinary meatus** (opening to exit body).
- Male: Passes through center of prostate before exiting through meatus.
- **External sphincter** (voluntary)
- **Note**: Normally, glucose and amino acids are reabsorbed into blood from nephron tubules. However, if there are excess amounts in the blood, then **renal threshold** occurs and these become part of urine.

Diagnostic Testing and Procedures

Catheterization: Tube inserted through urethra to bladder to remove or introduce fluids.

Dialysis: Artificial filtration of waste material from circulating blood.

Intravenous pyelogram (IVP): X-ray using dye to evaluate structure and function of kidneys.

Routine urinalysis: To check physical properties, specific gravity, and basic chemistry testing.

Urine culture: To ID pathogen(s) causing problem.

24-Hour urine collection: Testing urine sediment and content to diagnose various conditions.

Common Diseases and Conditions

Cystitis: Bladder infection; *Escherichia coli* most common cause.

Edema: Swelling due to fluid accumulation; symptoms of glomerulonephritis.

Glomerulonephritis: Glomerulus loses ability to be selectively permeable.

Hyperkalemia: ↑ Potassium level; electrolyte balance disorder.

Incontinence: Inability to retain urine; loss of urine upon coughing, sneezing, etc.

Polycystic kidney disease: Multiple cysts produced in kidney tubules, leads to kidney failure.

Pyelonephritis: Bacterial infection affecting renal pelvis.

Renal calculi: Kidney stones; contain calcium; more common in men.

Renal failure: Severe kidney damage, leads to failure; acute or chronic.

Wilms' tumor: In children ↓ 5; highest survival rate of all childhood cancers.

Word Roots

Root	Meaning
azot	Urea, nitrogen
cyst, vesic	Bladder = vesic, sac = cyst (holding fluid)
hydr	Water
lith	Stone, calculus
meat	Meatus
nephr, ren	Kidney
noct	Night
olig	Scant, few
pyel	Renal pelvis

Your Notes

Reproductive System

Functions	Cells, Tissues, Organs
FEMALE	**FEMALE**
1. Produce ova (singular = ovum) 2. Provide favorable environment for fetus to grow 3. Give birth to and feed newborn 4. Produce female hormones	1. Ovaries 2. Fallopian tubes 3. Uterus 4. Vagina 5. Vulva 6. Breasts
MALE	**MALE**
1. Produce sperm 2. Deposit sperm into female reproductive system 3. Produce male hormone	1. Scrotum and testes 2. Epididymis 3. Vas deferens 4. Seminal vesicles 5. Ejaculatory ducts and prostate gland 6. Cowper's (or bulbourethral) glands 7. Male urethra and penis

Organization—Female

Ovaries

Two glands manufacturing ova; secrete estrogen and progesterone.

Fallopian Tubes

- Curl around top of each ovary and connect to top corner of uterus to transport ova to uterus.
- Fertilization by sperm occurs here.

Uterus
Hollow, muscular; contains and nourishes developing embryo and fetus.

- Top of uterus called **fundus,** upper 2/3 called uterus.
- Lower 1/3 called **cervix.**
- Inner wall called **endometrium.**

Vagina
Muscular tube; leads from uterus to outside of body.

- Inner layer has rugae cells for expansion.
- Surrounded and partially covered by **hymen.**
- **Three functions**
  1. Lower end of birth canal.
  2. Receives the male organ and sperm.
  3. Provides passageway to outside for menstrual flow.

Vulva
Collective term for external genitals.

- Mons pubis: fatty tissue over pubic bone.
- Labia majora (vulval lips): enclose and protect urethral and vaginal openings, hair on outside.
- Labia minora: provides further protection.
- Clitoris: erectile tissue similar to penis, covered by prepuce.
- Skene's (urethral) and Bartholin's (vaginal) glands: secrete mucus and lubricating fluid.

Breasts
Mammary glands that produce milk.

Organization—Male

Scrotum and Testes
Testes suspended in sac of loose skin (scrotum).

- Before birth testes move from abdomen cavity to scrotum.
- Testes produce sperm.

Epididymis

Attached to side of each testis.

- Sperm mature and are stored here.

Vas Deferens

Tubes leading from epididymis to seminal vesicles.

Seminal Vesicles

- Secrete fructose-rich fluid; mix with sperm passing through vas deferens.

Ejaculatory Ducts and Prostate Gland

Ducts: Inside "donut-hole" of prostate; vas deferens and seminal vesicles join here

Gland: Secretes thin alkaline fluid; added to semen (60% of semen)

- Protects sperm from acids as it passes through urethra.

Cowper's or Bulbourethral Glands

- Secrete alkaline fluid (5% of semen).

Urethra and Penis

Urethra: 20 cm long, extends from ejaculatory tubes to tip of penis

Penis: Contains erectile tissue

- For copulation and urination.
- Becomes engorged with blood and firm when stimulated.
- Allows for female vaginal entry where sperm is ejaculated.
- Glans penis: tip, slightly wider than rest of penis.
- Prepuce (foreskin): extends over glans.

Additional Information

Apgar scoring system: Initial assessment of newborn; five signs are checked and scored—heart rate, respiratory rate, muscle tone, reflex irritability, and color.

Braxton-Hicks contraction: Irregular and occurs frequently in last month before labor.

Chadwick's sign: Thickening of vagina and development of purplish color in vagina and cervix.

Embryo: Name given through 8 weeks of development.

Fimbriae: Finger-like projections on fallopian tubes, produce a pulling action on ovum.

Gestation: Period of pregnancy—fertilization to birth.
Goodell's sign: Softening of the cervix, 5–6 weeks after fertilization.
Menarche: Initial onset of female menses, usually occurs between 9 and 15 years of age.
Menopause: Cessation of menstruation, usually around the ages of 48 to 50 years.
Menstruation (menses): Nonpregnancy shedding of endometrial lining, every 28 days.
Mitosis: One cell beginning to multiply through division; name of process.
Nagle's rule: Estimated date of confinement (or delivery); EDC or EDD.
Parturition: Technical term used for process of labor and delivery.
Placenta: Forms on uterine wall and joined to fetus by umbilical cord.
Quickening: A women's initial awareness of the movement of the fetus within her uterus; usually occurs between 18 and 20 weeks gestation.
Zygote: First cell; when sperm head unites with nucleus of ovum.

Diagnostic Testing and Procedures

Female

Amniocentesis: Needle insertion into amniotic sac to remove fluid for analysis.
Colposcopy: Visual examination of vaginal wall and cervix for abnormal cells.
Cryotherapy (cauterization): Freeze/burn technique, destroys abnormal cervix area cells.
D & C (dilation and curettage): Dilate cervix and scrape walls of uterus.
Mammogram: X-ray of breasts.
Pap smear (Papanicolaou test): Scraping of cervix and vagina, test for abnormal cell growth.
Tubal ligation: Fallopian tubes are severed, knotted, or blocked; result is sterilization.

Male

Circumcision: Surgical removal of foreskin (prepuce) of penis.
PSA (prostate-specific antigen): Test checking protein level released by prostate.
Vasectomy: Removal or knotting vas deferens; result is sterilization.

Common Diseases and Conditions

Female

Cystocele: Outpouching of bladder, protrudes into vagina; may cause urinary urgency.

Eclampsia (toxemia of pregnancy): ↑ BP, edema, protein in urine; untreated causes death.

Ectopic pregnancy (extrauterine): Implanted fetus outside of uterus; requires surgery.

Endometriosis: Endometrial tissue outside uterus; causes pain, cysts and tumors.

PID (pelvic inflammatory disease): Widespread bacterial infection of reproductive organs.

Placenta previa: Placenta blocks birth canal by attaching to lower uterine wall.

PMS (premenstrual syndrome): Symptoms of anxiety, bloating, irritability, headache, depression.

Infant

Cleft palate: Palatine bones improperly closed; passage between mouth and nasal cavities.

Down's syndrome: Extra chromosome (usually no. 21); causes mild to severe mental retardation.

PKU (phenylketonuria): Defective enzyme, cannot oxidize phenylalanine; can cause brain damage.

Spina bifida: Defect exposes spinal column; common in lumbar region.

Male

Benign prostatic hypertrophy: Enlargement of prostate, common if over 50 years.

Cryptorchidism: Failure of testes to descend into scrotum before birth.

Epididymitis: Epididymis inflammation; pain on urination, pain and swelling of scrotum.

Hydrocele: Accumulation of fluid within testes.

STDs

AIDS: Marked decrease in immunity; caused by HIV; no cure.

Chlamydia: Most common STD; from *Chlamydia trachomatis*; can cause female PID (pelvic inflammatory disease).

Condyloma: Wart growths on external genitalia; can cause cervical cancer.

Gonorrhea: Genital mucous membrane inflammation from *Neisseria gonorrhoeae.*

Herpes Genitalis: Viral; painful fluid-filled vesicles on genitals; can cause cervical cancer.

Syphilis: Infectious, chronic; results in lesions (chancres) on any organ or body part.

Trichomoniasis: Genitourinary parasitic infection; can result in female vaginitis.

Word Roots

Root	Meaning
arche	First, beginning
colp, vagin	Vagina
culd	Cul-de-sac
episi, vulv	Vulva
gynec, gyn	Woman
hyster, metr, uter	Uterus
mamm, mast	Breast
men	Menstruation
oophor	Ovary
salping	Fallopian tube
andr	Male
balan	Glans penis
epididym	Epididymis
orchid, orchid, orch, test	Testis
vas	Vessel, duct

Your Notes

Think you got all that?

Test yourself using your enclosed CD-ROM!

Notes

Notes

Gathering Patient Information

History

Components

- Presenting problem: Reason for visit
  1. CC (chief complaint).
  2. Signs (objective findings): Observed, test results, examination results.
  3. Symptoms (subjective findings): Patient provides information (e.g., pain scale 1–10).
  4. Give opportunity for child to express in their own words.
- Past and present diseases and medical problems: includes pregnancies and births (e.g., three children, one set of twins, two spontaneous abortions: G, no. of pregnancies; P, live births; Ab, abortions).
- Allergies and other peculiarities (anatomic abnormalities).
- Past surgery and injuries.
- Social history: alcohol, drugs, sexual orientation.
- Mental health: past and present.
- Family history: causes of death, diseases.

Common Medical Record Abbreviations

Abbreviation	Meaning
ALL	Allergy
BM	Bowel movement
bx, bi	Biopsy
CA	Cancer
CC or cc	Chief complaint
CNS	Central nervous system
CXR	Chest x-ray
DNR	Do not resuscitate
Dx	Diagnosis
ENT	Ears, nose, throat

Continued

Common Medical Record Abbreviations—cont'd

Abbreviation	Meaning
Ex, CPX, PE	Exam, examination
FH	Family history
f/u	Follow-up
GI	Gastrointestinal
HPI	History of present illness
Hx	History
N/O	No complaints
PERRLA	Pupils equal/round/reactive to light
PH	Past history
PT	Physical therapy
Px	Prognosis
R	Respiration
ROM	Range of motion
ROS	Review of systems
Rx, Tx	Treatment, prescription
SH	Social history
SOB	Shortness of breath
Sx	Symptoms
UA	Urinalysis
VS	Vital signs
WNL	Within normal limits
w/o	Without

Vital Statistics

Vital signs and height, weight.
Mensuration (measurements): Height, weight.

Vital Signs (Temperature, Pulse, Respiration, BP)

Useful in assessing present health of patient.
Can be compared with later readings to trace progress/course of disease.
Assist in diagnosis of disease.
Establish variation of normal range for a patient.

Temperature (Adults)		
Site	**Avg. in °F (Fahrenheit)**	**Avg. in °C (Celsius)**
Oral: under tongue in mouth	98.6	36.8
Rectal (R): rectum	100(R)	37.8(R)
Axillary (A): in armpit area (least accurate)	97.6 (A)	36.4 (A)
Tympanic (T): eardrum (quick/easy) **Adults:** Pull ear up and back **Children:** Pull ear down and back	100 (T)	37.8 (T)

Pyrexia: Fever
Febrile: Describes patient with fever

- Causes for ↓ body temperature:
  1. Blood loss
  2. Fainting
  3. Fasting
  4. Dehydration
  5. CNS injury

Pulse

- Measure using gentle pressure to artery against bone at site, infants require stethoscope.
- Rate: no. of heartbeats felt.
- Rhythm: tempo.

- Volume: strength.
- Indirect measure of cardiac output.
- Do not use thumb to measure—it has a pulse.
- Adult, 60–100 beats per minute; child, 70–120 beats per minute.
- Common pulse sites are:
  1. Apical: Lower left corner of heart; requires stethoscope; for infants
  2. Temporal: Over temporal bone at side of face
  3. Carotid: Side of neck, next to trachea
  4. Brachial: Within the bend of the elbow
  5. Radial: On the thumb side of the inner wrist
  6. Femoral: Groin
  7. Popliteal: Posterior to knee (check for circulation)
  8. Dorsalis pedis: Top of foot, medially (check for circulation)

Arrhythmia: Irregular beat.
Bradycardia: Slow, regular beat, ↓ than 60 per minute.
Bruit: Sound made by blockage in carotid artery.
Extrasystole: Right after normal beat, an extra heart contraction.
Pulse oximetry: Clips on finger or earlobe; measures % of oxygenated hemoglobin (Hgb); assesses status of pneumonia, bronchitis, emphysema, asthma patients; 95% or ↑ is normal.
Pulse pressure: Difference between systolic and diastolic reading; gives tone of arterial walls (↑ 50 or ↓ 30 mm Hg is abnormal).
Tachycardia: Rapid, regular beat, usually ↑ than 90 beats per minute.

Respiration

- Adult, 12–20 breaths per minute (count chest risings); child, 18–30 breaths per minute.
- Ratio of respirations to pulse rate, 1:4; evenly spaced, moderate depth, quiet.

Dyspnea: Difficult or painful breathing.
Eupnea: Normal breathing.
Exhalation: Lungs deflate, diaphragm rises to assist lungs.
Hyperpnea: Rapid, deep breathing.
Inspiration: Lungs fill, diaphragm moves down to allow expansion.
Tachypnea: Rapid breathing.

Blood Pressure: Arterial Pressure

- Measuring force of blood against artery walls.
- Common site is brachial artery: inside elbow of arm.
- Left arm gives slightly ↑ reading.
- ↑ With age; measured in mm Hg (millimeters of mercury).
- First sound is systolic; last sound is diastolic.

Diastolic: As left ventricle refills with blood; 60–80 mm Hg.
Korotkoff's sounds: Sounds between first and last sounds.
Sphygmomanometer: Used to measure BP.

- Dial: Registers pressure (mm Hg).
- Cuff: Regulates flow of blood through blood vessels.
- Pressure bulb: Used to pump air into cuff; inflate cuff 20 mm Hg above point that radial pulse disappears.
- Control valve: Controls release of air from cuff.

Systolic: Made as left ventricle contracts, sends blood into arteries; adults, 80–120 mm Hg.

- Do not use thumb on stethoscope bell—it has a pulse.

Vision Testing

- If measured as 20/30, means the smallest line patient sees at 20 feet is seen by normal eye at 30 feet.
- If measured as 20/40-1, means the smallest line patient sees at 20 feet is seen by normal eye at 40 feet minus 1 letter in line.

Color Blindness

Ishihara color number plate identification.
Green and red color blindness more common.
Occurs in ↑ number of males.

Infant Information

Newborns

- Receive first **Hepatitis B** immunization.
- BP 60–96/30–62 approximate range.
- 98.2°F (A) temperature average.

Apgar Score

- Measures: Appearance (color), pulse, grimace (reflex to stimuli), activity (muscle tone), respiration.
- Measured 1 and 5 minutes after birth, scored 0, 1,or 2; ↓ scores need attention.

Infants

- Head circumference measurement: just above eyebrows and top of ears (widest measure); performed until 36 months old.
- Pulse (apical): 100–160 beats per minute (use stethoscope, measure for 1 full minute, document as number and "AP" (apical).

Denver II Developmental Screening Test

- Screens gross and fine motor skills, personal skills, development.
- Administered periodically between 1 month and 6 years old.

Toddler

- Walks independently at approximately 12 months.
- Receives first **Hepatitis A** immunization at 12–23 months.

Examination

Auscultation: Listening to body sounds using stethoscope.

Inspection: Visual examination of patient (size, shape, symmetry, abnormalities, skin color and condition.

Manipulation: Moving body parts to assess range of motion.

Palpation: Touching skin surface and/or add some pressure to feel underlying organs to assess texture, temperature, movement, shape.

Percussion: Listening to body sounds by tapping body areas to assess resonance of appropriate organs, body cavities (e.g., lungs).

Romberg balance test: To assess muscle abnormalities.

- Patient stands with feet together, eyes closed.

Equipment

Common Instruments for Physical Examination

Ishihara color number plate: Tests for color blindness.

Nasal speculum: To check structures of nose in adults.

Ophthalmoscope: To check health of eyes; "red reflex" indicates good health.

Otoscope: To examine inner structures of ear.

Pen light: To check pupil response to light; to check nasal passages; tongue; mouth.

Percussion hammer: To check reflexes (neurological evaluation).

Pinwheel: To check touch sensation.

Pupil tonometer: Tests for glaucoma.

Snellen chart: Most often used to test vision; patient stands 20 feet (6 m) from chart.

Sphygmomanometer: To check BP.

Stethoscope: Used for auscultation.

Tape measure: Compare measurements of limbs, circumference of infant head.

Thermometer: To check temperature.

Tongue depressor and laryngeal mirror: To check mouth and throat.

Tuning fork: Used to assess hearing; size C most commonly used.

Vaginal speculum: To check structure of vagina.

Your Notes

Special Equipment

Instruments—Terms and Functions

Term	Instrument/Function
Cutting	Scissors, scalpel
Grasping/clamping	Hemostat, forceps, clamp, needle holder
Probing/dilating	Speculum, scope, probe, retractor, dilator
Laser	Converts light to intense beam used to vaporize tissue
Suture (verb)	To sew a wound, bring edges together (approximate)
Suture (noun)	Material used to sew

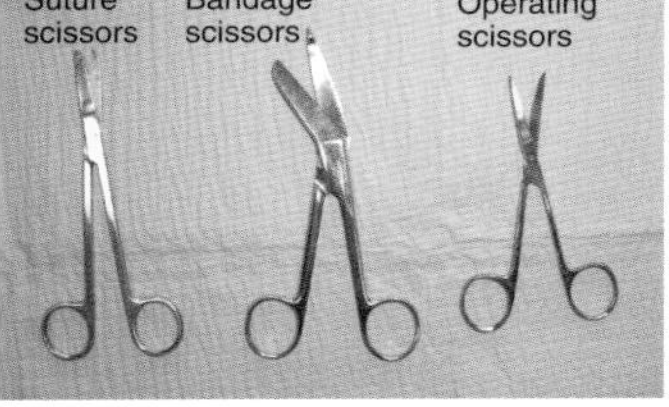

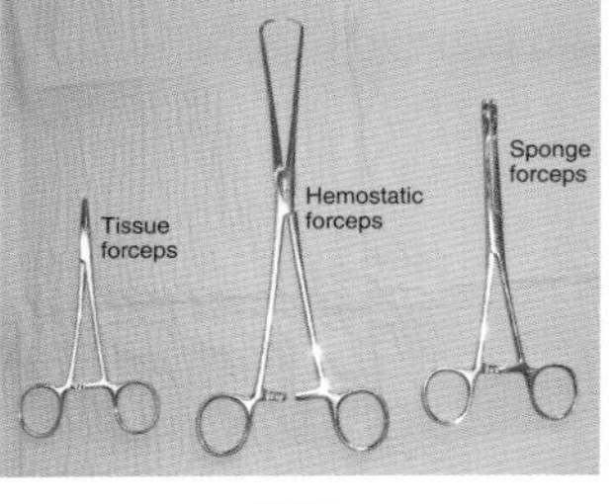

Asepsis

Surgical Asepsis

- When gloving, setting up, and maintaining sterile tray for:
  1. Suture removal
  2. Dressing change
  3. Urinary catheter insertion
  4. Minor laceration closure
  5. Sterile solution pouring
  6. Local infection incision and drainage (I&D)
  7. Culture collection
  8. Sterile technique used in all invasive procedures (venipuncture, parenteral administration, etc.)
     - Mantoux tuberculin skin test (a positive result shows area to be red, raised, hard).

Guidelines for Surgical Asepsis

- A 1-inch border around the sterile field is considered contaminated.
- Hold sterile items above waist; below the waist is considered contaminated.
- Always face the sterile field and never reach over the field.
- Place items in center of field.
- If you must leave the field, place a sterile towel over the field.
- Never cough or sneeze over sterile field.
- Try not to spill anything on the field.
- If a sterile object comes in contact with an unsterile item, it is now considered contaminated and cannot be used.
- If in doubt as to the sterility of an item, **DO NOT USE**.
- If the sterile field has been broken, start all over with set-up.

Source: Brassington, MA Review Notes, p. 123; Philadelphia: F.A. Davis, 2006

Medical Asepsis

Used for:

1. Dermal patch application
2. Oral/rectal/tympanic temperature measurement
3. Venipuncture
4. Cerumen removal
5. Proctoscopy
6. BP measurement
7. Eye irrigation/instillation

Examinations and Set-Ups

- **Prepping the Patient**: Explain examination and ask patient if they need assistance.

Positioning and Gowning

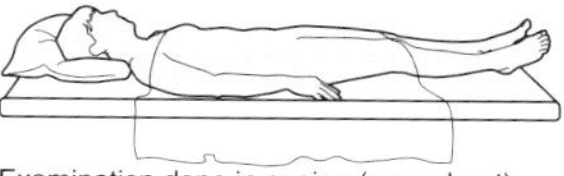

Examination done in supine (recumbent): breast, abdomen, arms, legs, head, neck,EKG

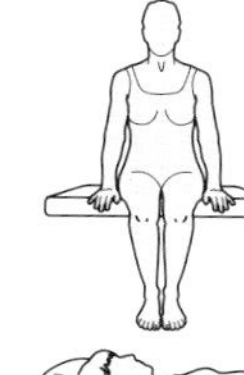

Examination done while sitting: head, neck, chest, heart, back, arms, lungs, knee/ankle reflexes

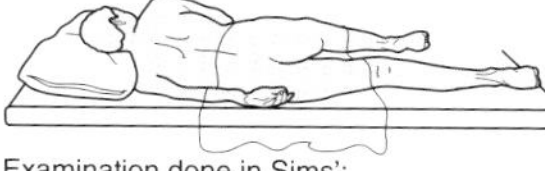

Examination done in Sims': flexsigmoidoscopy, anal

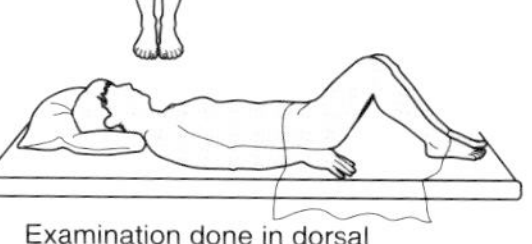

Examination done in dorsal recumbent: head, neck, chest, heart

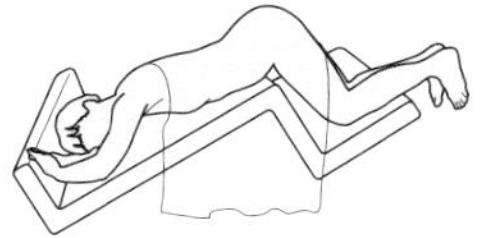

Examination done in protologic jack-knife: proctoscopic

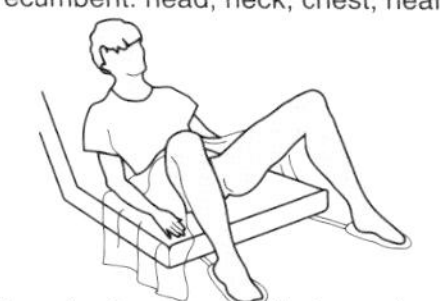

Examination done in lithotomy: female genitalia, endometrial biopsy

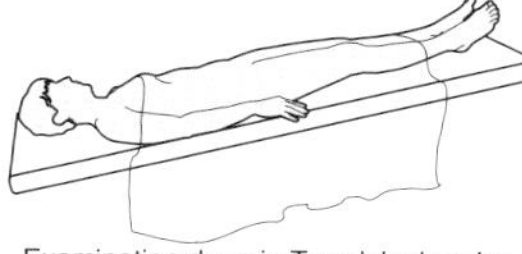

Examination done in Trendelenburg's: some surgical procedures, low BP, shock

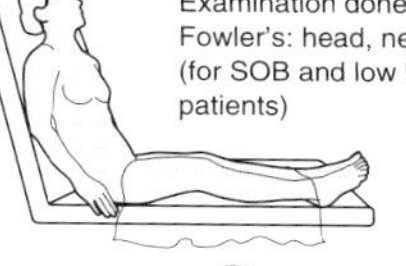

Examination done in Fowler's: head, neck, chest (for SOB and low back pain patients)

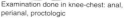

Examination done in prone: back, feet, musculoskeletal

Examination done in knee-chest: anal, perianal, proctologic

Emergencies and First Aid

Triaging

- Evaluating multiple patients and prioritizing for treatment (Tx).

Signs

- ↑ Bleeding, abnormal skin color, respiratory distress, convulsions, disorientation, unconsciousness, chest or severe pain, burns, ↑ or ↓ body temperature, bone fracture, deep wound.

Survey the Scene

1. **First**: (need to be done in this order) Is it safe to go into?
2. **Second**: Can you treat victims at site or remove them safely from it?
3. **Third**: Activate EMS (Emergency Medical System) if giving first aid.

Medical Office Equipment

- Cardiac code cart
- O_2 with mask delivery
- Cold packs
- Wound care kit
- PPE (personal protective equipment)
- Childbirth/delivery kit

ABCs of CPR

A: Check **a**irway
B: Look, listen, feel for **b**reathing
C: Check carotid for **c**irculation (pulse)

Second Assessments

Check for:

- Mental orientation.
- Level of consciousness (ask name, date).
- Take vital signs.
- Note skin color and moisture.
- Palpate for pain.
- Look for bleeding.

Burns

Type	Care
First degree: red, no blister	Immerse in cool water, apply sterile cool wet compress
Second degree: red, blistering	Immerse in cool water 1–2 hours, dry sterile dressing to cover
Third degree: full skin thickness, may involve muscle tissue	Thick dry sterile dressing to cover or dressing soaked in sterile saline solution if available, do not pull off adhered clothing, risk of infection and dehydration
Chemical	If powdered agent, try to brush off; if not, rinse copiously, then cover with sterile dressing

Myocardial Infarction (MI)

Signs and Symptoms	Care
Chest pain, left arm pain, jaw pain, sweating, indigestion, rapid respirations, nausea and vomiting	Activate EMS; get code cart and O_2, check ABCs if needed; vital signs, keep patient calm

Convulsions

Signs and Symptoms	Care
Jerking, spasmodic body movements, loss of consciousness	Activate EMS; protect head, maintain airway

Stroke—CVA (Cerebrovascular Accident)

Signs and Symptoms	Care
Slurred speech, confusion, paralysis to one side of body, unequal pupils	Activate EMS; maintain airway, check vital signs, keep patient calm

Syncope

Signs and Symptoms	Care
Unconscious due to $\downarrow$ BP or $\downarrow$ O_2	Place supine—head lower than heart, maintain open airway, apply cool compress to forehead, loosen tight clothing

Bleeding

Type	Care
Bleeding from limb, head, neck	Elevate injured part above heart if possible
All Types	**Care**
Severe bleeding	1. Direct pressure with sterile compress, add more as needed—don't replace used (disturbance to clotting process) 2. If needed, use indirect pressure on pulse point between wound and heart (slows bleeding process) 3. Life/death last resort is tourniquet application—note time of application

Shock

Signs and Symptoms	Care
Cool, pale, moist skin, ↓ BP, weak/rapid pulse, agitation, restlessness, dyspnea, weakness (may be due to severe blood loss)	Activate EMS; maintain airway, place in Trendelenburg position (if no head injury), check vital signs, keep patient warm

Common Types of Shock

- Traumatic: Loss of interstitial fluid (i.e., large burn areas).
- Hypovolemic (hemorrhagic): ↓ Blood volume.
- Cardiogenic: Impaired cardiac function.
- Septic: Infection that is spread by blood to all body systems.
- Neurogenic: Trauma to nervous system; fainting (blood vessels dilate, loss of tone, ↓ BP and heart rate.
- Anaphylactic: Severe allergic reaction (↓ BP, edema, tachycardia, dyspnea).
- Insulin.

Respiratory

Type	Care
Asthma: narrowing airways causing breathing difficulty, wheezing sound	Check ABCs; have patient sit upright, if possible; assist with inhaler; monitor O_2 with pulse oximeter; keep patient calm
Hyperventilation: leads to ↓ CO_2, dizziness, unconsciousness	Place paper bag over patient's nose and mouth, have them breath slowly, calmly
Choking: coughing audibly	Encourage to continue coughing
Choking: clutching throat, unable to produce sound	**Heimlich** maneuver ("bear hug" from behind, one hand covers balled fist below ribs and above navel, pull in with upward thrusts) to dislodge foreign object

Fractures

Types: Refer to Tab 4.
Care: Immobilize with splint, elevate (if possible), ice packs, slings for fractured clavicle, arms.

Poisoning

Type	Care
Inhaled, ingested, injected; chemical or natural	Activate EMS, call poison control for instructions, use PPE, check ABCs, check vital signs

Diabetic Conditions

Type	Care
Insulin shock: moist, pale skin, rapid heart rate, confused	Give food containing sugar that will be rapidly absorbed (orange juice, glucose gel)
Diabetic coma: dry, flushed skin, "fruity" breath, very thirsty, confused, rapid respiration	Activate EMS; provider must administer insulin

Physical Therapies

Gait

- Stance: Each leg supporting weight while other leg swings from behind to front.
- Swing: Each leg's motion from point of leaving floor to touching down.
- Observe stride length, balance, coordination, knee direction, foot direction.

Thermotherapy

Application of dry or moist heat for pain relief.

- ↓ Muscle spasms, localized swelling.
- ↑ Tissue repair.
- ↑ Infected area drainage.

Diathermy

Producing heat in body tissues by high-frequency currents.

- Used for arthritis, tendonitis.

Ultraviolet

Controlled lamp exposure therapy (for rickets, psoriasis, etc.).

Ultrasound

Uses water-soluble gel, high-frequency sound waves.

- Most common use of diathermy.

Cryotherapy

Application of dry or moist cold; used for:

- Vasoconstriction.
- Involuntary muscle contraction.
- Decreasing blood supply to area.
- Numbing effect on nerve endings.
- Controlling bleeding, swelling.
- ↓ Pain.

Massage

- Used to ↓ pain and tension.

Electric Muscle Stimulation

TENS (transcutaneous electric nerve stimulation) unit for orthopedics such as:

- Arthritis.
- Back injury, sports injury.
- Not for patients with cardiac disease or pacemakers because of electrical stimulation.

Traction

Part of body is pulled/stretched.

- Aligns bones, relieves vertebral bone compression.
- Reduces/relieves muscle spasms and shortenings.

Mobility Devices

- **Walkers:** Top of walker should be just below waist, same height as top of hip bone; elbows bend at 30° while using.
- **Crutches:** 1–1.5 inch below armpits; handgrips at top of hipline; stand on good leg, move crutches ahead of good foot.

Crutch Walking Patterns

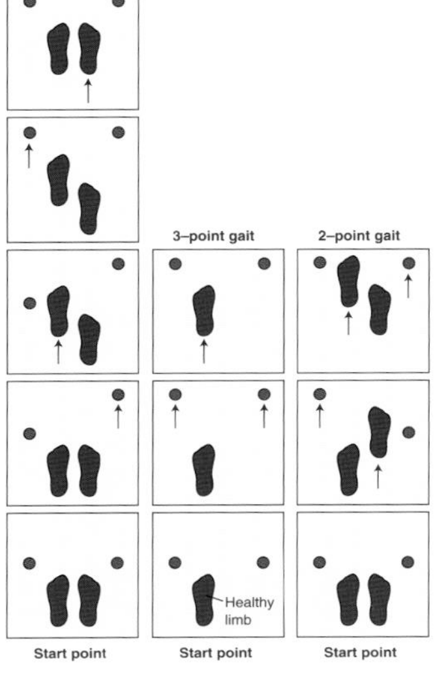

Nutrition

Diet Components

Basal Metabolic Rate (BMR)

- Energy used while fasting/resting to maintain vital functions.

Calorie

- Unit of heat energy.
- Amount of O_2 used.

Carbohydrates

- For energy; classified by complexity.
  1. A simple sugar (i.e., white bread, rice, potatoes, pasta).
  2. A complex plant food (i.e., most vegetable and fruit produce).

Proteins

- Build and repair body tissue.
- Composed of amino acids.

Fats

For energy and heat.

- Saturated: From animals.
- Unsaturated: Liquid at room temperature.
- Monounsaturated: Olives, avocados.
- Polyunsaturated: Nuts, seeds.

Food Group	Daily Recommendation
Grains: ↑st amount	At least 3 oz. of "whole" grain
Vegetables	Vary these, eat more dark green and orange
Fruits	Variety: fresh, frozen, canned, dried, ↓ juice
Dairy	Go for low-fat or no-fat
Meat and beans	Low-fat or lean meats, poultry, fish (bake, broil, grill), nuts, beans
Oils: ↓st amount	Fish, nuts, vegetables; ↓ solid fats (butter, shortening) no trans fats

Vitamin	Function
A	Fat-soluble, beta carotene, prevent night blindness
E	Fat-soluble, anticoagulant
D	Fat-soluble, for calcium absorption, ↓ rickets and osteomalacia
K	Fat-soluble, for blood clotting, ↓ hemorrhage
C	Water-soluble, ↓ scurvy, heals wounds, infection protection
B complex	Water-soluble, metabolism, hemoglobin formation

Mineral	Function
Calcium	Builds bone, cardiac function, muscle contraction, blood coagulation
Chloride	Body pH and fluid balance
Phosphorus	Metabolism of protein, calcium, glucose
Sodium	Body pH balance, muscle contraction control, kidney regulates level
Potassium	Protein synthesis, pH balance, heartbeat regulation
Magnesium	Builds bone, metabolism, enzyme activities
Zinc	For growth, healing, sense of taste, glucose tolerance
Iron	Hemoglobin component needed for O_2 transport through body

Your Notes

Think you got all that?

Test yourself using your enclosed CD-ROM!

Notes

Pharmacology

- Study of drugs and their origin, nature, properties, and effect on living organisms.
- Drugs are used to give an individual a "within normal range" test result.

Drug Laws

Pure Food and Drug Act (1906)

- First drug law passed in US.
- For consumer quality.
- Set US standards for making each drug; USP/NF.

Federal Food, Drug and Cosmetic Act of (1938)

- FDA established by Department of Health and Welfare.
- Regulations to prevent adulteration (tampering).
- Accurate labels with generic name included.
- New products must be FDA approved.
- Warning labels used.
- Rx and non-Rx drugs must be shown to be effective and safe.
- Drug utilization review required.

Controlled Substances Act (1970)

- Established by DEA through Department of Justice.
- Drug controlled by Rx requirement due to abuse and addiction danger (depressants, stimulants, psychedelics, narcotics, anabolic steroids).
- On-site responsibilities:
  1. Maintain 2-year inventory of controlled drug transactions.
  2. All prescribers register with DEA and obtain DEA registration number.
  3. Securely store all Rx forms at facility.
  4. Keep a current drug reference book available at all times.
  5. Keep controlled substances locked securely (double-locked).

Drug Names

Generic/Official
- Common/general name given when drug is first produced.
- Not protected by trademark and less costly.

Trade/Brand
- Upon FDA approval, manufacturer gives it this name.

Chemical
- Scientific molecular formula of drug (long and complicated).

Rights and Uses

Rights in Drug Administration	Drug Uses
Right dose: Amount of drug	**Treatment:** Relieves disease/disorder symptoms
Right drug: Check label three times (on removal from storage, while preparing, upon return to storage)	**Diagnostic:** Tests for allergies (antigen sera), radiographic studies (dye injection)
Right route	**Palliative:** For patient comfort; no cure; relieves pain or other symptoms
Right time	**Preventative/prophylactic:** Stops disease or condition from occurring
Right patient	**Replacement:** Treat illness/condition (hormones, vitamins, etc.)
Right documentation: Patient name; date and time of administration; drug and dosage given; route used and complications; any adverse reactions and reasons for not administering	**Therapeutic/curative:** Healing

Prescription (Legend) Components

- Written by MD, filled by pharmacist.
- Indicates medication needed and contains all directions for pharmacist and patient.
  1. Name of drug
  2. Dosage
  3. When drug is to be given
  4. How it is given
  5. How many times it is given
  6. Date of the order
  7. Signature of MD who wrote it

Superscription: Describes prescription.
Subscription: Number of doses dispensed and directions given to pharmacist.
Sig. (signature): Tells pharmacist what to write on label (patient instructions).

Drug Action Factors

Absorption

- Route and time it takes for drug to work after taken.
- Rate drug passes from intestines into bloodstream and amount passing into bloodstream.
- Injection bypasses this stage.
- Two effects: **localized** (lotion, ointment); **systemic** (overall effect on body).

Distribution

- Drug leaves blood and passes into tissues spaces and cell bodies.
- May pass across **blood-brain barrier** (regulates selection, degree and rate of absorption into brain tissue) or placenta into fetus.

Metabolism (Biotransformation)

- Drug breakdown within liver to another chemical.
- Usually results in inactivation of drug.
- Sometimes converted to active form after liver absorption.

Elimination

- Route by which drug is eliminated.
- Excretion in urine is most common.
- Small amounts excreted in saliva, sweat, stool, breast milk, breathing, tears.

Drug Actions

Actions

- Describes cellular changes due to drug usage.
- Technical info.

Cautions

- Conditions that require close observation for specific side effects.

Contraindications

- Conditions for which drug administration is improper/undesirable.

Factors Altering Usual Effects

Tolerance: Reduced responsiveness to drug.

1. Could be inherited or acquired due to usage over length of time.

Cumulation: Accumulation of drug in body resulting in toxicity.

1. Drug has much greater effect and toxic side effects.
2. Usually due to lack of elimination between administrations.
3. Other factors are weight, age, sex, environment, psychologic, genetics, allergies.

Indications

- Conditions for which a drug is meant to be used.

Interactions

- Listing of drugs or foods that will alter drugs effect; should not be given at time of drug therapy.

Synergism: Occurs when combining drugs.

1. The presence of one drug increases intensity or prolongs duration of another drug's effect.
2. Two drugs may produce same type of effect.

Potentiation: A synergistic action when only one of the drugs exerts a greater action due to an inactive drug for the first drug's treatment usage (eg, an anticoagulant may be potentiated by use of an anti-inflammatory agent).

Antagonism: Occurs when presence of 1 drug decreases the intensity or shortens duration of another drug's effect.

1. One drug cancels the effect of another (e.g., antibiotics associated with birth control pill failure).

Local

- Acts on limited area where it is administered; external.

Side Effects and Adverse Reactions

- List of possible unwanted effects, unpleasant or dangerous aside from desired effect.

Common side effects (unintended)

1. Drowsiness, dizziness, headache.
2. Osteoporosis, hives, diarrhea, nausea and vomiting, rash, alopecia.

Other effects

1. Ototoxicity, tinnitus, photosensitivity.
2. Nephrotoxicity.

Systemic

- Transported through bloodstream and carried to one or more body tissues.
- General effect.

Toxic Effects

- Poisonous
- Result of idiosyncrasies, or single overdose, or accumulation in blood levels over time

Drug Forms

Capsules: Two-part containers; shell dissolves in GI tract and inside are drug-imbedded powder or beads.

Caplets: Shaped like capsule but consistency of tablet.

Elixirs: Solution containing sugar, alcohol, water.

Emulsions: Fine droplets of fat globules in water (homogenized milk).

Liniments: Drugs mixed with oil, soap, water, or alcohol used externally on skin to produce warmth.
Lotions: Suspension or emulsion preparation used externally on skin.
Ointments: Semisolid salve with fatty base; applied externally to skin.
Spirits: Solution containing alcohol.
Suppositories: Semisolid form designed to melt after insertion; used rectally, vaginally, or in urethra.
Suspensions: Particles of drug scattered within a liquid, not dissolved.
Syrups: Liquids containing sugar (e.g., ipecac).
Tablets: Compressed powder; various shapes, colors; some **enteric**-coated, **buccal,** sublingual, scored.
Tincture: Solution of drug(s) dissolved in alcohol with or without water.
Transdermal patch: Adhesive patch/disc to skin in area drug needed.

Drug Routes of Absorption

Transdermal Patches

- Slow time release of drugs (estrogen, nicotine) through skin.

Oral

- Convenient, safe, relatively inexpensive; most taken 1–2 hours p.c. (after meals).

Mucous Membrane

- Local uses: eye drops, nasal sprays, rectal suppositories for constipation, vaginal.
- Systemic uses: rectal suppositories for vomiting, sublingual for angina, inhalation for lower respiratory tract.

Ophthalmic

1. Eye ointment: tip allows dispensing of small stream into bottom eyelid.
2. Eye drops: place in center of lower conjunctival sac.

Otic (ear) drop instillation

1. For adults: pull pinna up and back.
2. For children under 3 years old: pull lobe down and back.

Rectal: Patient should be in Sims' position for insertion.
Sublingual: Under tongue.

Inhalation: Inhaled.
Urethral: Inserted.

Topical

- Used on skin, eyes, ears; not absorbed by outer skin layers.
- For skin itching, inflammation, skin infections.

Parenteral

- Ways drug administered by injection; surest, fastest method.
- ↑ Risk of overdosing (OD).
- Effectiveness determined by site blood supply.
    - **IV** (intravenous) is instantaneous, **IM** (intramuscular) faster than **SC** (subcutaneous), **ID** (intradermal).

Injections

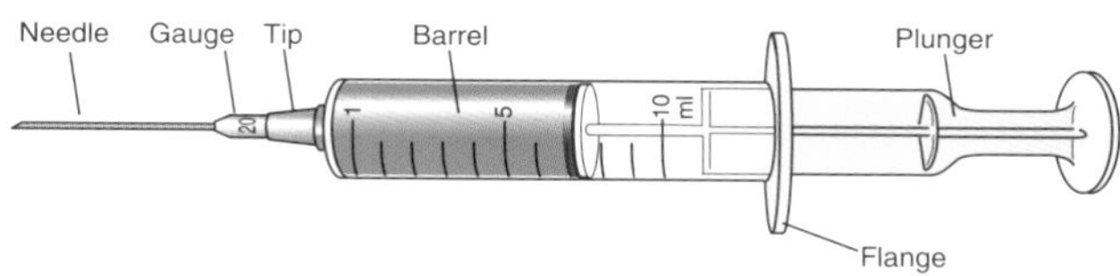

Gauges

- Determined by size of needle lumen (diameter of opening).
- The higher the gauge number, the smaller the lumen.

ID Injection

- Bevel up, do not aspirate (PPD—purified protein derivative tuberculin test).

SC Injection

- Grasp skin, form 1-inch fold, aspirate, inject slowly.
- For insulin injection: roll vial between palms to evenly mix, do not shake, do not massage after injection (also true in administering Imferon, heparin).

IM Injection

- Stretch skin taut, aspirate, inject slowly, cover site, massage.
- For **adults,** preferred site for deep IM is dorsogluteal site (upper outer buttock quadrant).
- For **infants,** Vastus lateralis—anterolateral area of thighs (upper lateral quadrant of thigh).
- **"Z-Track" injection**: Pull skin 1.5 inch away from injection site, insert at 90° angle, dart-like, aspirate, inject slowly, wait 10 seconds before withdrawing, remove needle at same angle, release skin, no massage.

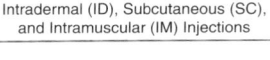

Intradermal (ID), Subcutaneous (SC), and Intramuscular (IM) Injections

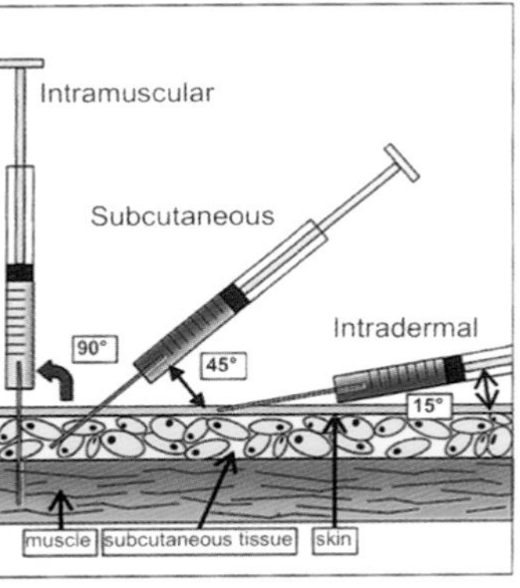

Courtesy of Ehren Myers and Tracy Hopkins, MedSurg Notes, F.A. Davis Company, 2004

Immunizations

Recommended Immunization Schedule for Persons Aged 7 Through 18 Years—United States 2009

Range of recommended ages

Certain high-risk groups

Catch-up immunization

<table>
<tr><th>Vaccine / Age</th><th>7–10 years</th><th>11–12 years</th><th>13–18 years</th></tr>
<tr><td>Diphtheria, Tetanus, Pertussis</td><td></td><td>Tdap</td><td>Tdap</td></tr>
<tr><td>Human Papillomavirus</td><td></td><td>HPV (3 doses)</td><td>HPV series</td></tr>
<tr><td>Meningococcal</td><td>MCV</td><td>MCV</td><td>MCV</td></tr>
<tr><td>Influenza</td><td colspan="3">Influenza (yearly)</td></tr>
<tr><td>Pneumococcal</td><td colspan="3">PPSV</td></tr>
<tr><td>Hepatitis A</td><td colspan="3">HepA series</td></tr>
<tr><td>Hepatitis B</td><td colspan="3">HepB series</td></tr>
<tr><td>Inactivated Poliovirus</td><td colspan="3">IPV series</td></tr>
<tr><td>Measles, Mumps, Rubella</td><td colspan="3">MMR series</td></tr>
<tr><td>Varicella</td><td colspan="3">Varicella series</td></tr>
</table>

Recommended Immunization Schedule for Persons Aged 0 Through 6 Years—United States 2009

Range of recommended ages | Certain high-risk groups

Vaccine / Age	Birth	1 month	2 months	4 months	6 months	12 months	15 months	18 months	19–23 months	2–3 years	4–6 years
Hepatitis B	Hep B	HepB			HepB						
Rotavirus			Rota	Rota	Rota						
Diphtheria, Tetanus, Pertussis			DTaP	DTaP	DTaP		DTaP				DTaP
Haemophilus influenzae type B			Hib	Hib	*Hib*	Hib					
Pneumococcal			PCV	PCV	PCV	PCV				PPSV	
Inactivated Poliovirus			IPV	IPV	IPV						IPV
Influenza					Influenza (yearly)						
Measles, Mumps, Rubella						MMR					MMR
Varicella						Varicella					Varicella
Hepatitis A						HepA (2 doses)				Hep A series	
Meningococcal										MCV	

Catch-Up Immunization Schedule for Persons Aged 4 Months Through 6 Years Who Start Late or Who Are More Than 1 Month Behind—United States 2009

The table below provides catch-up schedules and minimum intervals between doses for children whose vaccinations have been delayed. A vaccine series does not need to be restarted, regardless of the time that has elapsed between doses. Use the section appropriate for the child's age.

Vaccine	Minimum age for dose 1	Minimum interval between doses			
		Dose 1 to dose 2	Dose 2 to dose 3	Dose 3 to dose 4	Dose 4 to dose 5
Hepatitis B	Birth	4 weeks	8 weeks and at least16 weeks after first dose		
Rotavirus	6 wks	4 weeks	4 weeks		
Diphtheria, Tetanus, Pertussis	6 wks	4 weeks	4 weeks	6 months	6 months
Haemophilus influenza type B	6 wks	4 weeks if first dose administered at younger than age 12 months 8 weeks (as final dose) if first dose administered at age 12–14 months No further doses needed if first dose administered at age 15 months or older	4 weeks if current age is younger than 12 months 8 weeks (as final dose) if current age is 12 months or older and second dose administered at younger than age 15 months No further doses needed if previous dose administered at age 15 months or older	8 weeks (as final dose) This dose is only necessary for children aged 12 months through 59 months who received 3 doses before age 12 months	
Pneumococcal	6 wks	4 weeks if first dose administered at younger than age 12 months 8 weeks as final dose for healthy children, if first dose administered at age 12 months or older or current age 24–59 months No further doses needed for healthy children, if first dose administered at age 24 months or older	4 weeks if current age is younger than 12 months 8 weeks as final dose for healthy children, if current age is 12 months or older No further doses needed for healthy children if previous dose administered at age 24 months or older	8 weeks (as final dose) This dose is only necessary for children aged 12 months through 59 months who received 3 doses before age 12 months or for high-risk children who received 3 doses at any age	
Inactivated Poliovirus	6 wks	4 weeks	4 weeks	4 weeks	
Measles, Mumps, Rubella	12 mos	4 weeks			
Varicella	12 mos	3 months			
Hepatitis A	12 mos	6 months			

Catch-Up Immunization Schedule for Persons Aged 7 Years Through 18 Years—United States 2009

Vaccine	Minimum age for dose 1	Minimum interval between doses			
		Dose 1 to dose 2	**Dose 2 to dose 3**	**Dose 3 to dose 4**	**Dose 4 to dose 5**
Tetanus, Diphtheria/ Tetanus, Diphtheria, Pertussis	7 yrs	4 weeks	4 weeks if first dose administered younger than 12 months 6 months if first dose administered at age 12 months or older	6 months if first dose administered younger than 12 months	
Human Papillomavirus	9 yrs	Routine dosing intervals are recommended			
Hepatitis A	12 mos	6 months			
Hepatitis B	Birth	4 weeks	8 weeks and at least 16 weeks after first dose		
Inactivated Poliovirus	6 wks	4 weeks	4 weeks	4 weeks	
Measles, Mumps, Rubella	12 mos	4 weeks			
Varicella	12 mos	3 months if the person is younger than age 13 years 4 weeks if person is aged 13 years or older			

*Data courtesy of Centers for Disease Control. (**Note:** The CDC updates the immunization chart yearly; refer to the most current chart for further information.)*

Classifications

Analgesics

Trade Name	Generic Name	Used for/Actions
Acetaminophen with codeine		Also antipyretic
Endocet	oxycodone/APAP	Pain reliever, narcotic
Naproxen		Nonopioid pain reliever, NSAID (nonsteroidal anti-inflammatory drug), antipyretic
Novocaine (topical)		Numbing local topical area
Lidocaine 0.5% injection		Localized numbing
OxyContin	oxycodone	Chronic moderate/severe pain relief
Percocet, Roxicet	oxycodone/ acetaminophen	Pain reliever, narcotic
Ultram	tramadol hydrochloride	Moderate pain relief, non-narcotic

Anti-Allergy

Trade Name	Generic Name	Used for/Actions
Allegra	fexofenadine	Antihistamine
Atarax	hydroxyzine hydrochloride	Antihistamine, antiemetic
Clarinex	desloratadine	H1 histamine antagonist
Hydrocodone	hydrocodone bitartrate	Antitussive for nonproductive dry cough, narcotic
Zyrtec	cetirizine	Antihistamine, chronic idiopathic urticaria

Antibiotics

Trade Name	Generic Name	Used for/Actions
Amoxicillin		Anti-infective, systemic chronic/ acute
Amoxil	amoxicillin	Anti-infective, antiulcer, ENT infection
Augmentin		ENT, soft-tissue infection
Bactrim	trimethoprim, sulfamethoxazole	UTI (urinary tract infection), URI (upper respiratory infection), otitis media
Biaxin	clarithromycin	URI, skin infections
Cefzil	cefprozil	*Streptococcus* and *Staphylococcus* causing URI and skin infections
Cipro	ciprofloxacin	UTI, URI, bone/joint infection

Anticoagulants

Trade Name	Generic Name	Used for/Actions
Aspirin	aspirin or ASA (acetylsalicylic acid)	Blood thinner, analgesic, antipyretic
Coumadin	warfarin	Blood thinner

Anti-Arrhythmic

Trade Name	Generic Name	Used for/Actions
Dilantin	phenytoin	Anticonvulsant
Lanoxin	digoxin	Slows and strengthens heartbeat

Antidepressants		
Trade Name	**Generic Name**	**Used for/Actions**
Paxil	paroxetine hydrochloride	Also anxiety, panic disorder
Wellbutrin XL	bupropion hydrochloride	Depression
Zoloft	sertraline hydrochloride	Also obsessive-compulsive disorder

Antidiabetics		
Trade Name	**Generic Name**	**Used for/Actions**
Avandia	rosiglitazone maleate	NIDDM (non-insulin dependent diabetes mellitus) Type 2
Glucophage	metformin	NIDDM (non-insulin dependent diabetes mellitus) Type 2
Glucotrol XL	glipizide	NIDDM (non-insulin dependent diabetes mellitus) Type 2

Antifungals		
Trade Name	**Generic Name**	**Used for/Actions**
Diflucan	fluconazole	Oropharyngeal, vaginal and systemic candidiasis
Mycostatin	nystatin	*Candida* skin and mucous membrane infections

Antihypertensives

Trade Name	Generic Name	Used for/Actions
Accupril	quinapril hydrochloride	Hypertension, CHF (congestive heart failure)/ACE (angiotensin-converting enzyme) inhibitor
Cozaar	losartan potassium	Hypertension
Lasix	furosemide	Hypertension, CHF, diuretic for edema
Lotensin	benazepril hydrochloride	Hypertensive
Norvasc	amlodipine besylate	Hypertension, angina, Ca (calcium) channel blocker
Prinivil	lisinopril	Hypertension, ACE inhibitor, CHF
Toprol XL	metoprolol succinate	Hypertension, angina pectoris
Zestril	lisinopril	Hypertensive, ACE inhibitor, CHF

Anti-Inflammatories

Trade Name	Generic Name	Used for/Actions
Naproxen		Arthritis, dysmenorrhea
Celebrex	celecoxib	Pain associated with arthritis

Anti-Ulcer Agents

Trade Name	Generic Name	Used for/Actions
Prevacid	Lansoprazole	Active duodenal ulcer, gastric ulcer, erosive esophagitis
Prilosec	Omeprazole	Gastric and duodenal ulcers, gastroesophageal reflux disease (GERD)

Bronchodilators

Trade Name	Generic Name	Used for/Actions
Proventil HFA	albuterol	Bronchospasm associated with asthma, bronchitis
Aminophylline	theophylline ethylenediamine	Bronchospasm prevention and symptom relief
Epi-E-Zpen, Primatene Mist Suspension	epinephrine	Temporary bronchospasm relief due to asthma, anaphylactic reactions

Corticosteroids

Trade Name	Generic Name	Used for/Actions
Flonase	fluticasone	Seasonal allergic rhinitis
Nasonex	mometasone furoate	Steroid-dependent asthma, seasonal rhinitis

Hormones

Trade Name	Generic Name	Used for/Actions
Climara	estradiol	Contraceptive, HRT (hormone replacement)
Premarin	estrogen	Osteoporosis, menopausal symptoms
Synthroid	levothyroxine	Hypothyroidism, cretinism, myxedema
Humulin N insulin	isophane insulin, human rDNA	Hyperglycemia, IDDM (insulin dependent diabetes mellitus) Type 1

Hypnotics/Sedatives

Trade Name	Generic Name	Used for/Actions
Ambien	zolpidem tartrate	Insomnia
Lunesta	eszopiclone	Insomnia

Supplements/Replacements

Trade Name	Generic Name	Used for/Actions
Fosamax	Alendronate	Increase bone density
Levoxyl	Levothyroxine	Thyroid product
Klor-Con	Potassium chloride	Electrolyte supplement

Drug Schedule

Established due to danger of:

- **Physical dependence** (need for medication to relieve shaking, pain or other symptoms).
- **Psychologic dependence** (anxiety, stress, tension felt by patient if without medication).

Schedule I

Drugs with ↑ addiction potential, no medicinal use (heroin, mescaline, LSD).

Schedule II

Drugs with ↑ addiction potential, have medicinal use (cocaine, morphine, methadone, codeine, Nembutal, Percodan, Tylox).

Provider must have DEA number to prescribe, provider must sign prescription.

Prescription must be furnished to pharmacy within 72 hours.

If stored in office: must be locked, routinely counted, inventoried, dispensing record kept for 2 years.

Schedule III

Drugs with ↓ physical dependence, ↑ psychological dependence, limited amounts of cocaine, narcotics or amphetamine-like substances (barbiturates, amphetamine compounds, paregoric, Fiorinal).

Prescription handwritten, no DEA number required; up to 5 refills in 6 months.

Schedule IV

Drugs with ↓ abuse potential than III, mild tranquilizers and hypnotics.

Prescription written by MA or RN, but signed by MD, up to 5 refills in 6 months, refills by phone (diazepam, Librium, valium, Ambien).

Schedule V

Drugs require a written or oral prescription.

Orders and refills same as for schedule IV (↓ codeine level, Lomotil, Robitussin A-C).

Measurements

Metric System

Volume = liters (L)
1,000 milliliters (mL) = 1 L
Weight = grams (g)
1,000 milligrams (mg) = 1 g
1,000 g = 1 kilogram (kg)
Length = meters (m)
100 centimeters (cm) = 1 m

Unit(s)	Metric Prefix Term	Decimal Form
100 units	hecto	100
10 units	deka	10
1,000 units	kilo	1,000
One tenth of a unit	deci	0.1
One thousandth of a unit	milli	0.001
One millionth of a unit	micro	0.000001
One hundredth of a unit	centi	0.01

- To change from a larger unit to a smaller unit: × by 1,000 or just move decimal point 3 places to the right.
- To change from a smaller unit to a larger unit: ÷ by 1,000 or just move decimal point 3 places to the left.

Approximate Equivalents to Household Measures

Volume: 1 teaspoon (tsp) = 5 mL
1 tablespoon (tbsp) = 15 mL
1 ounce (oz) = 30 mL
1 cup (8 oz) = 240 mL
1 pint = 500 mL
1 quart = 1,000 mL, 1,000 cc (cubic centimeters; also cm^3)
Weight: 1 ounce = 30 g
16 ounces (oz) = 1 pound (lb)
2.2 lb = 1 kg
Length: 2.5 cm = 1 inch (in)

Temperature Conversion

- Formula to convert Fahrenheit (F) to Celsius (C): C = (F – 32) × 5/9
  First: Subtract 32 from the Fahrenheit temperature.
  Second: Multiply result by 5.
  Third: Divide result by 9.
- Formula to convert Celsius (C) to Fahrenheit (F): F = 9 × c + 32
  First: Multiply C by 9.
  Second: Divide result by 5.
  Third: Add 32 to result.

Dosing

Geriatric: Considerations are: metabolism, GI function, drug sensitivity, hydration, safest route, psychosocial changes, circulation.
Adults: Based on age (20–60 years old) and weight (avg. 150 lbs).
Children: Usually calculated on basis of mg of drug/kg of body weight.

Use of Proportion to Solve for X in Dosing Problem

The sequence used on left side of equals sign must be the same on the right
You know either both your means or extremes

Multiply the known means or extremes
Divide the answer by the one remaining known (an extreme or mean)

Example
4 mg : 50 lbs = X mg : 150 lbs
Both extremes are known; 4 and 150
Multiply them; 600
Divide by known mean; 50
X = 12 mg

Your Notes

Additional Abbreviations

Abbreviation	Meaning	Abbreviation	Meaning
aa	of each	**npo**	nothing by mouth
a.c.	before meals	**OD**	right eye
AD	right ear	**ophth**	instill in eyes
ad lib	as desired	**OS**	left eye
amt	amount	**otic**	instill in ears
aq	water	**OU**	both eyes
AS	left ear	**p**	after
AU	both ears	**p.c.**	after meals
b.i.d. or **BID**	twice a day	**per**	by, with
c	with	**po** or **PO**	by mouth
caps	capsules	**prn** or **PRN**	as needed
d/c or **DC**	discontinue	**q**	every
disp	dispense	**qd**	every day
dl, dL	deciliter	**qh**	every hour
elix	elixir	**q2h**	every 2 hours
emul	emulsion	**q6h**	every 6 hours
et	and	**q.i.d.** or **QID**	four times a day
fl	fluid	**qod**	every other day
h, hr	hour	**qs**	quantity sufficient
hs or **HS**	hour of sleep	**s**	without
K	potassium	**sig**	label
mcg	microgram	**ss**	one half
n	normal	**stat** or **STAT**	immediately
NaCl	sodium chloride	**t.i.d.** or **TID**	three times a day

More Vocabulary

Ampule: Prefilled small glass container holding sterile solution or powder; has scored neck; designed for 1 use only.

Aspirate: Part of injection process; pulling back on hypodermic plunger to assure the needle is not in blood vessel (no blood should be present in barrel; failure to do so may deliver IM or SC injection to be delivered IV).
Average dose: Most effective with minimum toxic effect.
Buccal: Drug form to be placed between cheek and gum, do not chew.
Cartridge-needle unit: Disposable; holds premeasured medication.
Cumulative dose: After repeated medication dosing, this is total amount present in the body.
Dispense: Prepare and give out a medication to patient.
Divided dose: A smaller measured portion given at shorter intervals.
Enteric-coated: Drug form designed to bypass stomach and then dissolve in intestine.
Initial dose: The first dose.
Maintenance dose: Amount needed to remain at therapeutic level in bloodstream.
Maximum dose: Safest, largest amount that can be given.
Medication unit: Expresses potency of drugs too varied in their potency (insulin).
Minimum dose: The smallest amount that will still be effective.
Pharmacodynamics: Study of drugs and their actions on living organisms.
Pharmacokinetics: Study of drug actions and metabolism within the body.
Prescribe: Recommend/order therapeutic treatment or use of a drug.
Solution: Liquid homogeneous preparation; contains 1 or more substances.

- **Solute:** Dissolved substance.
- **Solvent:** Liquid in which solute is dissolved.

Toxic dose: Amount causing signs and symptoms of drug toxicity.
Vial: Prefilled small glass container holding sterile solution or powder; rubber stopped for needle entry.
Viscosity: Liquid thickness and stickiness.
Wheal: Slight elevation of skin; the result of ID injection.

Think you got all that?

 **Test yourself using your enclosed CD-ROM!**

Notes

Pathogens

Any microorganism that causes disease.

Chain of Infection

Reservoir host

Can be:
- insect
- animal
- person

Exits host by:
- break in skin
- body orifice

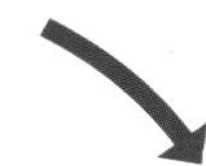

Transmission

Movement to new host by:
- sneeze
- contaminated materials, food, water, or hands

Portal of entry

Movement to new host by:
- blood supply (vein)
- skin break (cut)
- oral, nasal, eye, ear, rectal, or genital opening

New host

Susceptible because:
- weak immunity
- virulent pathogen

Infectious Agents

Bacteria Types

Aerobe (requires O_2 to survive).

Anaerobes (will die with O_2).

- Prefixes
  - Chains = strepto-
  - Pairs = diplo-
  - Clusters = staphylo-

Cocci (round); singular **coccus**

- Causes pneumonia, strep throat, gonorrhea

Bacilli (rod-shaped); singular: **bacillus**

- Causes: tuberculosis (TB), tetanus, UTI, whooping cough

Spirilla (spiral); singular **spirillum**

- Causes syphilis, Lyme disease

Stained Slides

Gram-positive bacteria (purple): Botulism, diphtheria, pneumonia, rheumatic fever, staph infection, tetanus, streptococcal throat.

Gram-negative bacteria (pink): Gonorrhea, meningitis, UTI, cholera, pertussis, plague, typhoid fever, dysentery.

Fungi: Eukaryotes

- Larger than bacteria.

Tinea: superficial infection; causes:

1. Athlete's foot (tinea pedis)
2. Ringworm
3. Thrush (oral yeast)

Parasites

- Harm and live on/in human body.
- Identified in urine, tissue biopsy, fluids.
  1. Worms (helminths): round, whip, tape, pin.
  2. Single-celled (protozoa): malaria, dysentery.

Virus

- Small microscopic pathogen (i.e., herpes, HIV, hepatitis, rubella, mumps).

Blood-borne viral infections:

- Disease lives in and transmits through blood.

Hepatitis Types	
A	Acute infective: caused by hepatitis A virus (HAV); transmitted by fecal/oral contamination
B	Most common; caused by HBV; infection is transmitted through contaminated serum, plasma, needles, and entry through all entry portals
C	Non-AB; transmitted by blood transfusion or needle sharing
D	Delta; occurs in hepatitis B patients; transmitted by needle sharing and sex
E	Acute; mostly outside U.S.; transmitted by fecal-contaminated water or food

HIV: Transmitted acutely:

- Blood-to-blood and sexual contact
- May be present in all body fluids
- 70% of the infected acquire **AIDS**

Stages of HIV Infection	
Stage 1	Acute HIV infection, HIV carrier
Stage 2	Asymptomatic latency (may be years)
Stage 3	AIDS-related complex (ARC)
Final stage: AIDS	May have Kaposi's sarcoma (skin lesion CA), *Pneumocystis carinii* (severe pneumonia), patient has no immunity

Asepsis (Without Infection)

Handwashing

Most important single method of asepsis.

Medical Aseptic Handwashing

- Keep hands lower than forearms (water flows into sink instead of back onto arms).
- With water running, dry hands with clean, dry paper towels, then turn off faucets using clean, dry paper towel.

Surgical Aseptic Handwashing

- Use sterile scrub brush.
- Hands and forearms are washed.
- Hands are held above elbows (water cannot flow from arms onto washed areas).
- Sterile towels are used instead of paper towels.

Antiseptics

- Used to cleanse infective agents from human tissue, use outward circular motion from incision site for 2–5 minutes.

Sanitization

- Scrubbing process for cleansing instruments.
- Removes debris and blood.
- Prepares instruments for disinfection by chemicals, steam, heat, gases.

Disinfection

- Used on instruments/countertops; i.e., glutaraldehyde (Cidex), chemical germicides, household bleach (sodium hypochlorite).

Sterilization

- Destroys all microorganisms by dry heat, steam heat, chemical, or gases.
  1. **Gas**: for large equipment (e.g., beds); used in hospitals.
  2. **Dry heat**: For instruments prone to corrosion.
  3. **Chemical**: For heat-sensitive equipment.
  4. **Steam heat**: Autoclave—most common method in medical offices.
     - Operate with distilled water.
     - Wrap instruments (hinged instruments wrapped in open position).
     - Steam temperature must be 250°F–254°F.
     - For effective sterilization, 20–40 minutes.
     - Begin timing when indicators show recommended temperature and pressure.
     - Maximum shelf life for a sterile pack is 30 days.

Laboratory Safety

Standard (Universal) Precautions

- Treat all blood and body fluids as contaminated.
- Protect patients from you; protect yourself from patients.

Personal Protective Equipment (PPE)

- Sterile or nonsterile gloves, lab coat, shoe covers, gown.
- Protective eyewear, mask, face shield.

Environment Safety

- Employee training, employer accidental exposure plan, use of hazard warning labels where needed, MSDS (material safety data sheets) for hazardous agents.
- Puncture-proof sharps containers, biohazard bags, eyewash stations.

Specimen Collection, Handling and Quality Control

Collection

Before Collection

- Review requisition slip and confirm patient's proper test preparation.
- Hand wash before/after each procedure.
- Wear gloves when appropriate.
- All hazardous waste disposed of in biohazard labeled bag/puncture-proof container.
- Micro- and venipuncture sites are cleansed with alcohol, use spiral technique working from inside to outer edges and air dried or dried with sterile gauze.
- Use sterile collection containers and/or equipment.
- Label container: patient's name, date, time of collection, specimen source, your initials.
- Incubate culture plates with agar side up, moisture droplets will not fall on growing surface.

Handling

- Store specimen according to instructions; refrigerate, separate blood components, etc.
- Avoid contaminating specimen or self.
- Transport disease-causing microorganism using agar (sheep's blood) as medium: ensures nutrition for microorganism.

Quality Control

- Specimen collected for pathologic testing is placed in formalin preservative; for microbiologic culturing Tx as sterile as possible and no exposure to formalin.
- Giving patient procedure performance instructions, give verbal and written instruction, and confirm their understanding of procedure steps.
- Clinical employees given refresher lab procedure training each year.
- Check expiration dates of collection containers, tubes, swabs, reagents, etc., before use.
- Procedure manual describes test process, proper result reporting and documentation.
- Calibrate laboratory instruments and verify calibrations at least every 6 months.
- Perform and document control testing each day on appropriate tests; document action when errors occur.
- Perform and document equipment maintenance; cleaning, adjusting, part replacement.

Pulmonary Function Test (PFT)

Evaluates lung volume and capacity.

Spirometry

- Evaluates lung capacity.

Preparation

1. Stand straight
2. Inhale slow deep breath
3. Expel all air quickly

Forced vital capacity (FVC): Greatest volume of air expelled in a rapid, forced expiration after inhaling as deep as possible.

- **Test result**: Below 80% is abnormal.
- **Contraindications to testing**: Recent MI, angina, serious medical condition, smoking/eating meal within 6 hours of test, viral infection or illness in past 2 weeks, use of some medications may affect test results.

Hematology: Analysis of Blood

Blood

Whole Blood

- Total volume is 55% plasma, 45% formed elements.

Plasma

- 90% water, 9% protein, 1% fats, carbohydrates, gases, waste products, clotting factors, and minerals.
- After centrifuging, plasma is highest in tube.

Formed Elements

- Erythrocytes; leukocytes; platelets (thrombocytes).
- Cells formed mostly in red bone marrow.

Micropuncture

- Select (great) middle or ring finger of non-dominant hand; on infants use underside of outer edge of heel.
- Cleanse with alcohol pad, allow to dry/wipe with sterile gauze pad.
- Puncture should be no deeper than 2.4 mm (0.1").
- Wipe away first droplet of blood because it contains more tissue fluid.

Whole Blood Testing

Hemoglobin (Hb or Hgb)

- Normal range: men, 14–18 g/dL; women, 12–16 g/dL.

Hematocrit (Hct)

- Approximately 3 × Hb measurement ± 3.
- Normal range: men, 42%–52%; women, 37%–47%.
- Duplicate Hct results should not vary by more than 2% of each other.
- Layers in spun (or centrifuged) Hct (from top to bottom): plasma, "buffy coat," packed RBCs.

Bleeding Time

- Evaluates the blood's ability to clot; normal range 2–7 minutes.

Blood Typing

ABO antigens and Rh factor (D antigens): Agglutination points to type.

1. Type O: no agglutination
2. Type O-negative: universal donor
3. Type AB-positive: universal recipient

ESR (Erythrocyte Sedimentation Rate or "Sed Rate")

- Measured as millimeters per hour (mm/h)
- Determines degree of inflammation in body
- Wintrobe and Westergren method used

Glucose

- Chemistry test; normal range, 70–110 mg/dL.

GTT (glucose tolerance test)

- Timed
- Routine at 6 months of pregnancy
- Tests carbohydrate metabolism; preparation is:
    1. Eat ↑ carb diet for 3 days
    2. Fast 8–12 hours before
    3. May have a little water
    4. First draw to start should be ↓ 150 mg/dL, then given glucose orally
    5. Half hour later, draw blood and urine each hour as MD prescribes

Cholesterol

- Chemistry test, normal results are:
  1. Total < 200 mg/dL
  2. LDL (low-density lipoprotein) < 130 mg/dL
  3. HDL (high-density lipoprotein) > 35 mg/dL

Venipuncture

- Most commonly performed for hematologic testing.
- Most common site is median cubital vein; cephalic (thumb side on forearm) and basilic veins and back of hand veins.

Needles

- The ↑ the gauge number, the ↑ risk of hemolysis.
- Use 19–23 gauge.
- For butterfly needle, 21–25 gauge.
- Insert at approximately15° angle.
- Steady and quick, insert ½ to ¼ inch.
- Tourniquet in place in ↓ 2 minutes.

Collection Tubes

- Adults, usually 3–10-mL tubes.
- Children, usually 2–4-mL tubes.
- Tube color determines tube content.
- Invert tubes five to 10 times to process specimen with additive in tube.
- EDTA (ethylenediaminetetraacetic acid) is the preferred anticoagulant for hematology studies.

Recommended Order of Draw

Color	Tube Contents	Used to Test For
First: yellow	Sodium polyanethol-sulfonate (SPS)	Blood cultures
Second: red	None	Chemistry, blood banking, immunology
Third: light blue	Sodium citrate	Coagulation studies
Fourth: red/black (tiger/mottled)	SST: serum gel separator, clot activator	Chemistry and immunology tests requiring serum
Fifth: green	Heparin	Chemistry, electrolyte studies, arterial blood gases
Sixth: lavender	EDTA, an anticoagulant	Hematology studies
Seventh: gray	Potassium oxalate or sodium fluoride, anticoagulants	Blood glucose, lactic analysis

Serology (Immunology)

Serology

- Study of serum.
- Measure of antigens or antibodies present (hormones, vitamins, drugs).
- Presence of antibodies measured by a **titer**.
- Most chemistry tests performed on serum.

If Found in Serum	Disorder/Disease Indicated
BUN (blood urea nitrogen)	Kidney disorder
AST (aspartate aminotransferase)	Liver disease; mononucleosis (mono), damaged cardiac or skeletal muscle
ADH (antidiuretic hormone)	Brain tumor
Acetone	Diabetic metabolic ketoacidosis
Amylase	Pancreatic disorder, drug toxicity
ALT (alanine aminotransferase)	Liver disorder

Immunology

- Study of sensitivity and allergy by reaction between antigen and antibody.

Hormone detection: pregnancy (human chorionic gonadotropin; HCG)
Virus detection: infectious mononucleosis (Epstein-Barr virus), HIV
Bacteria detection: duodenal ulcers: 90% (*Helicobacter pylori*), Lyme disease (infected tick), strep throat (*Streptococcus pyogenes*)

Urinalysis

Collection

- 95% water, 5% waste products; average adult produces 1,250 mL/day (1.25 L).
- Must be room temperature and well mixed before testing.
- Refrigerate if not analyzing immediately (within 1 hour).

Specimen Types

Random

- Most common sample type
- Routine screening
- Collect 3 oz or more

First Morning Specimen

- Highest solute concentration
- Highest specific gravity

Fasting Sample

- Second morning specimen
- A must for diabetic monitoring

Clean-Catch Midstream

- Best for bacterial culture
- Keep inside of container sterile and as free as possible of bacteria surrounding urethra

24-Hour

- For quantitative analysis
- Calcium, potassium, creatinine, urea nitrogen, protein, lead levels
- Begin collection after first morning void

Analysis

Physical Examination

Color: pale straw to dark amber; other color indicators are:

Color	Possible Causes
Colorless	Drinking excessive amounts of water
Red	Blackberry, cranberry, beets, blood (kidney/bladder infection, CA (cancer), trauma)
Neon yellow	B-complex vitamin, excess riboflavin (B_2)
Orange	Pyridium (drug to treat bladder infection)
Dark yellow	Dehydration, early sign of liver problem
Brown	Beans (especially fava), rhubarb, old disintegrated blood clots
Blue	Methylene blue (drug ingredient for bladder spasm and discomfort)

Clarity: rate from transparent to turbid.

Specific gravity: density measurement compared to distilled water.

- Normal range: 1.005–1.030.
- Measured by urinometer or refractometer.

Odor

- Fruity indicates diabetes
- Foul indicates infection
- Ammonia scent indicates ↑ concentration of bacteria from sitting at room temperature too long

Chemical Examination

Reagent pads

- On strips dipped into sample.
- Pads react by changing color.
- Timed measurements.
- Measures pH (normal range, 4.5–8.0) and the following:

Abnormal Reagent Pad Result	Indicates
Albumin (protein)	UTI
Ketone bodies (acetone)	↑ Fat diet, severe diabetes mellitus, starvation, body wasting
Bilirubin (degenerated RBCs)	Points to liver damage
Urobilinogen (converted bilirubin)	Points to heart, liver, spleen disease
Blood	Kidney damage, urinary tract disease
Nitrate	Microorganisms, specimen left out ↑ 2 hours, bacteria create nitrite in vivo
Glucose	Possible diabetes mellitus, above renal threshold

Microscopic Examination

- After centrifuging, pour off **supernatant**.
- Set up wet mount to examine urine sediment.
- Normal findings are: WBCs < 5 normal, hyaline casts, crystals.

Abnormal Urine Crystals	Indicates
Cystine: six-sided	By a genetic defect; can cause mental retardation
Tyrosine needle and Leucine spheroid	Severe liver disease
Cholesterol	Severe urinary tract infections

Abnormal Urine Casts	Indicates
↑ No. of hyaline casts	Kidney disease or heavy exercise
WBC casts	Pyelonephritis
Granular casts	Heavy exercise or renal disease
RBC casts	Glomerulonephritis
Renal tubular epithelial casts	Ischemia
Waxy casts	Severe renal disease

Microscope

- Move microscope by grasping arm and supporting weight at base.

Oculars

- Contain magnifying lens, usually magnifies 10 times (10× lens).

Objectives: three mounted on a swivel base

1. Each has magnifying lens
2. Two objectives (10× lens is low power and 40× lens is high power) are dry (air between objective and prepared slide)
3. One objective (100× lens) is oil-immersed (oil drop touches lens and prepared slide)

Stage

- Prepared slide placed here and held in place with metal clips.
- Opening in stage allows light passage to slide.

Condenser

- On substage, directs concentrated light through slide.

Iris (Diaphragm)

- Controls amount of light used by opening and closing.

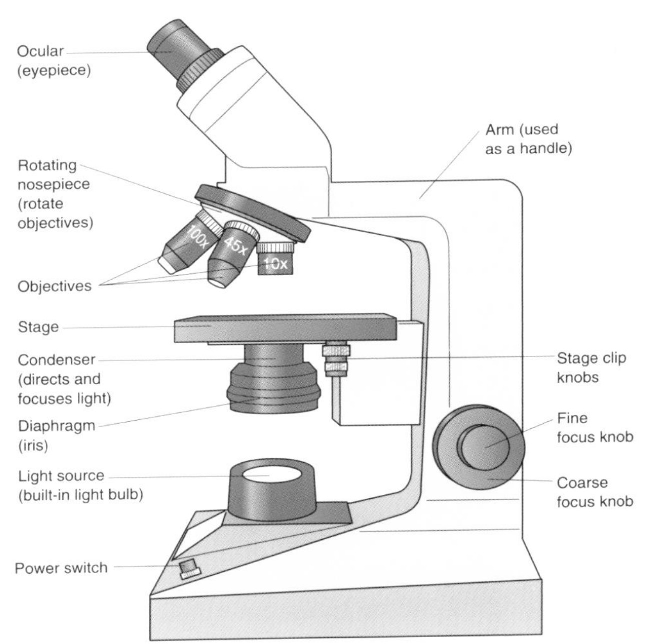
Ocular
(eyepiece)
Arm (used
as a handle)
Rotating
nosepiece
(rotate
objectives)
100x
45x
10x
Objectives
Stage
Condenser
(directs and
focuses light)
Stage clip
knobs
Diaphragm
(iris)
Fine
focus knob
Light source
(built-in light bulb)
Coarse
focus knob
Power switch

Cardiac Cycle and ECG (EKG)

Cardiac Cycle

- Complete cycle, 0.8 seconds.
- Regulated by electrical impulses transmitted through heart wall tissues.

Normal Rate of Rhythm (RR)

- 60–100 beats per minute.

Complete Cycle

- Heart contracts (**depolarization**) then relaxes (**repolarization**).
- Atria first contract, followed by ventricles.
- This action moves blood out of heart into body.

SA (Sinoatrial) Node

- Picks up electrical impulse and triggers cardiac cycle.
- Responsible for atrial contraction.
- Triggers AV node.

AV (Atrioventricular) Node

- Briefly delays impulses from SA node.
- This keeps ventricles from contracting too soon.
- Allows atria to completely contract, gets all blood out and into ventricles.
- Fires at 46–60 beats per minute.

Bundle of His

- Triggered by AV node.
- Carries impulse to **left and right bundle branches and** eventually to **Purkinje fibers.**
  - These three are responsible for ventricle contraction.
- Ventricle cells fire at 20–40 beats per minute.

Final Phase

- Heartbeat relaxes (**repolarization**).

Electrical Conduction of the Heart

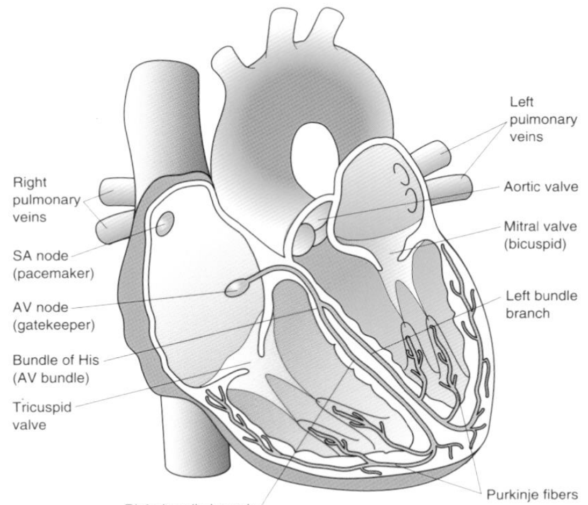

12-Lead EKG (ECG)

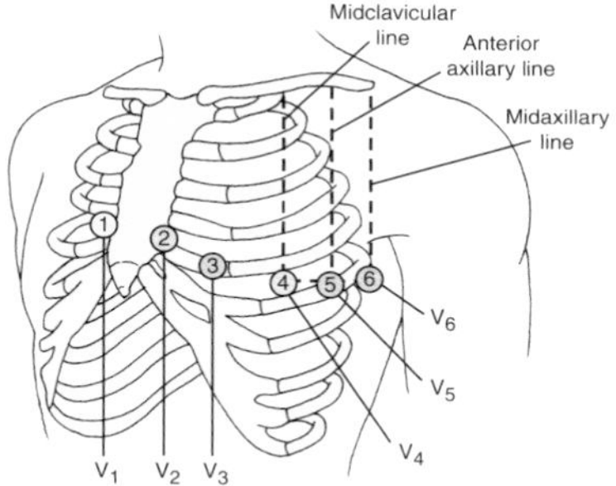

Lead	Placement
V_1	Below left clavicle, just lateral to the midclavicular line
V_2	At the fourth rib to the left of the sternal border
V_3	Below right clavicle, just lateral to the midclavicular line
V_4	Fifth rib at anterior axillary line
V_5	At manubrium sterni
V_6	At the sixth rib on the midclavicular line

- A 12-lead EKG records three **bipolar** leads, three **unipolar** leads, six chest leads (**precordial**).
- Ensure patient's comfort before performing EKG.
- Six electrodes are placed on the upper torso, one electrode is placed on each limb.
- Place electrodes on fleshy part of upper arms and lower legs to decrease possibility of muscle voltage (**artifacts**).
- Holter monitor: five leads and used to record cardiac activity over 24-hour period.

Reading the EKG

One Full Cardiac Cycle

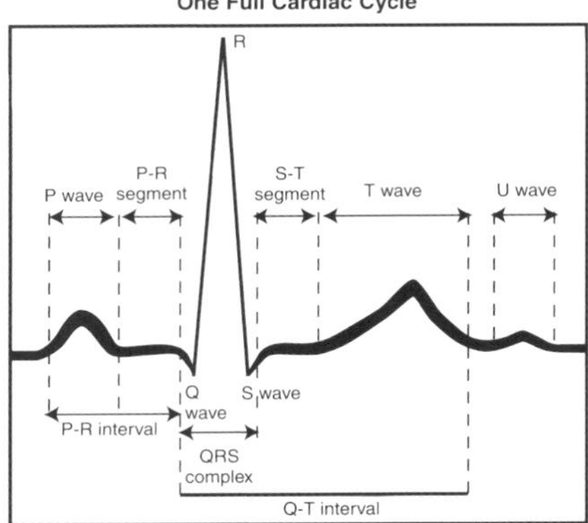

P Wave

- Represents depolarization of atria.
- Measures atrial activity.

P-R Interval

- Time it takes electrical impulse to be conducted through atria and AV node.

QRS Complex

- Represents depolarization of ventricles.

T Wave

- Represents heart repolarization (relaxing).
- Rounded, usually ↑ than P wave.

EKG Paper

- An EKG standardization mark is 10 mm high.
- If baseline is off-center, need to adjust stylus position.
- EKG paper rolls out at 25 mm (1 inch) per second.

- Each line on paper grid is 1 mm apart.
- Each small box: 0.04 seconds.
- Each large box (5 small boxes across): 0.20 seconds.
- 0.8 seconds (a cardiac cycle) is represented as two small boxes long.
- RL (right leg) not displayed because it is the ground electrode.

Artifacts

Somatic tremor: Body muscle movement (spasm).
Electrical interference: Machine not well grounded or close to other electrical device.
Baseline interruption: Broken lead or no longer in place.
Wandering baseline: Poor skin connection or loose electrode.

Radiology

Common Types

CT (or CAT): computed axial tomography

- Rapid, thin detailed tissue planes.

MRI (Magnetic Resonance Imaging)

- Views internal structures (soft and hard tissues).
- No preparation needed.
- Metal objects cannot be worn or imbedded (no mascara, no pacemaker).

IVP

- Views of urinary structures.
- Uses iodine injection.
- Preparation: clear liquids day before, then NPO 8 hours before.

KUB (Flat Plate)

- **K**idneys, **U**reters, **B**ladder.
- Used to diagnose disease.

Cholecystography

- Uses contrast medium.
- Preparation: no food/drink 12–14 hours before.
- Uses contrast medium.

Colonoscopy

- Views entire colon.
- Preparation: clear liquid diet, bowel stimulants 24 hours before.

Barium Enema (Lower GI Series)

- To view lower portion of GI system.
- Uses barium.
- Preparation: drink clear liquids day before.

Barium Swallow (Upper GI Series)

- To view upper portion of GI system.
- Uses barium.
- Preparation: NPO 8 hours before.

Ultrasound (US)

- Ultrasonic waves produce image of deep body structures.
- Preparation: may require full bladder.

Positron Emission Tomography (PET Scan)

- Produces color images to assess activity and structures.
- Uses radioisotope injection.

Radiation Therapy

- Treats disease (shrinks cancer tumors).

Positioning

- **AP (anteroposterior)**: Patient supine, beam guided from front to back.
- **PA (posteroanterior)**: Patient prone, beam guided from back to front.
- **RL (right lateral)**: Patient lying on right side, beam guided from left side to right side.
- **LL (left lateral)**: Patient lying on left side, beam guided from right side to left side.
- **Oblique**: Patient lying at angle, beam guided through body (left posterior or left anterior oblique, right posterior or right anterior oblique).

Safety

Monitored dosimeter: Worn by those present during x-rays.

Lead shields: To cover organs not needed to x-ray (especially reproductive organs).

Pregnancy alert: Patient asked if pregnant; if so notify radiologist before x-ray.

Equipment: Inspected, maintained properly.

Lead aprons: For use by staff: if not behind protective shield during procedure.

Proper disposal: In preferred and labeled containers for radioactive materials.

Your Notes

Think you got all that?

Test yourself using your enclosed CD-ROM!

Notes

Notes

Psychology Theories

Maslow's Hierarchy of Needs

5th Need

Self-actualization, Fulfillment

Self-realization, sense of fulfillment in accomplishments

4th Need

Self-esteem, Status

Sense of self-worth and pride, growth oriented

3rd Need

Love and Social

Sense of belonging, social interaction, self-respect

2nd Need

Security and Safety

Physical safety and security

1st Need

Physical survival

Food, water, air, shelter

To Understand Someone's Motivation

- First, see level of need being threatened.
- Generally, you may not progress to next level until previous-level needs have been met.

Elisabeth Kübler-Ross' Stages of Death and Dying

1st: Denial	A buffer against the harsh reality, deny existence of problem
2nd: Anger	Rage, unfairness of situation, "why me?"
3rd: Bargaining	Spiritual, bargaining with God and/or healthcare workers
4th: Depression	Quiet grieving, facing loss of self, some withdrawal from others here
5th: Acceptance	Resigned to fate and planning for it

- Stages are not mutually exclusive, may overlap, repeat; may skip stages.
- Stages enable us to understand all grieving people: facing death, loved one loss, amputation, various body function loss, preferred lifestyle loss, economic loss, divorce.

Psychological Disorders

Anxiety

- Tension, worry, apprehension; moderate to severe.

Obsessive-Compulsive Disorder

- Behavior involving repetitive thoughts and actions.

Panic Attack

- Sudden extreme anxiety; rapid heartbeat and breathing, sweating.

Phobias

1. **Agoraphobia:** Fear of being in public places outside of home.
2. **Acrophobia:** Fear of high places.
3. **Claustrophobia:** Fear of being confined in any space.
4. **Hydrophobia:** Fear of water.
5. **Social anxiety disorder:** Fear of being judged/criticized while performing routine behaviors in front of others at social gathering.

Post-traumatic Stress Disorder

- Long-lasting.
- Response to physical/psychological trauma.

Mood

- Emotions affecting ability to function and/or causing psychological discomfort.

Bipolar Disorder ("Manic Depression")

- Extreme mood swings, highs and lows.

Dysphoria

- Depression and unrest without apparent cause.

Major Depression

- Profound loss of all hope.

Seasonal Affective Disorder (SAD)

- Seasonal depression.
- Mostly fall and winter.

Other Disorders

Anorexia Nervosa

- Severely restricted calorie intake.
- Result of ↑ fear of weight gain.

Autism

- Severely impaired social/communications skills.
- Preoccupation with inner thoughts.

Bulimia Nervosa

- Repeated episodes of binge eating followed by purging.

Confabulation

- Cover-up used for memory gaps.
- Patient fabricates ideas and uses inappropriate words.

Dementia

- Mental deterioration due to brain disease.

Hypochondriasis

- Belief one has various diseases.
- Problems do not resolve after reassurances that disease is not present.

Paranoia

- Show of persistent persecutory delusions or delusional jealousy.
- May exhibit schizophrenic symptoms.

Schizophrenia

- Psychosis.
- Display delusions, hallucinations, disorganized speech and behavior.

Somatization

- Recurrent and multiple body (any organ system) complaints with no physical basis.

Tourette's Syndrome

- Uncontrollable motor tics, facial tics, verbal grunts and use of profanity.

Your Notes

Professionalism

Appearance

- Appropriate dress.
- Personal hygiene.

Conduct

- Treat each patient with dignity and respect.
- Exercise diplomacy.
- Be courteous.
- Speak in a professional manner.
- Do not initiate or comment negatively regarding another medical office professional when you are speaking to patients.
- Do not speak of patients outside of office environment.
- Be honest (admitting your mistakes to supervisor); this ensures ↑ quality care and ↓ chance for litigation.

Verbal and Nonverbal Communication

- Communication should strive to fulfill the "Five Cs":
  1. Clear
  2. Cohesive
  3. Complete
  4. Concise
  5. Courteous

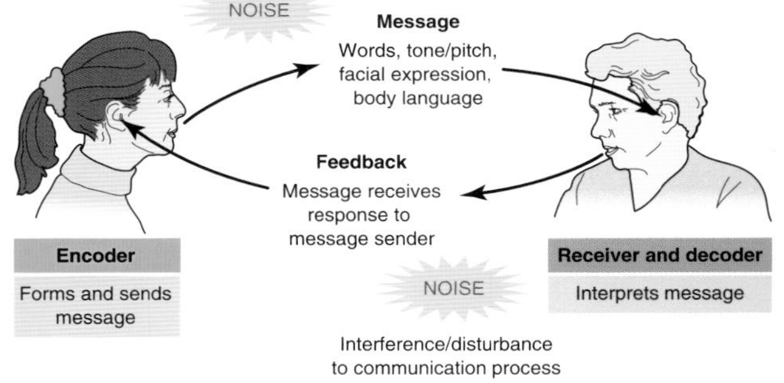

Communication Terms

Accountability: To be responsible for actions and words.
Body language: Most of what is said is communicated this way.
Closed-ended questions: Requires **yes** or **no** or a **number.**
Effective use of silence: Patient uses time to think before responding; may add new information.
Empathy: Putting oneself in another person's place in order to realize their feelings.
Feedback: Either verbal or nonverbal; response to communicating message.
Non-judgment: Should be evident in facial expression, body language, and responses made.
Open-ended questions: Requires more than yes or no; tell me about yourself.
Paraphrasing/restating: Telling messenger what you heard, using your own words.
Perception: Being aware of your own feelings and feelings of others.
Reflecting: Repeating what is heard using open-ended statements that patient must complete.

Nonverbal Communication

Body Language (Kinesics: Study of Body Movements)

- Tapping foot: restlessness.
- Drumming fingers: indifference, apathy.
- Head scratching: uncertainty, bewilderment.

Eye Contact
Face-to-Face
Gesturing

- Hand/arm movement.
- Emphasizes ideas and emotions.
- Enhances message communicated.

Leaning Body

- Forward toward person shows interest.

Posture

- Erect: suggests self-confidence.
- Slumped: suggests sadness, no confidence.

Proximity

- Observing space boundaries (comfort zone) between patient and caregiver.
  - "Personal space": 1.4–4 feet.
  - "Social space": 4–12 feet.
  - "Public space": 12–25 feet.

Touch

- Can show sensitivity and concern if used on someone who is receptive.

Forms of Listening

Active Listening

- Give your full attention.
- Nodding.
- Smiling.
- Asking questions.
- Taking notes.

Evaluative Listening

- Provides immediate response and opinion.
- Avoiding selective hearing.

Passive Listening

- No required feedback.
- As an audience member.

Special Circumstances

Children

- At their level, speak to them eye-to-eye.
- Always speak calmly, gently, using short simple sentences that are age appropriate.
- Always state the truth.
- Allow privacy from adults (especially adolescents) during assessment if desired.
- Encourage questions.

Geriatric

- Ensure patient's comfort, privacy, and safety in examination room.
- Face the patient when speaking.
- Speak clearly, do not shout.

Hearing Impaired

- Communicate in quiet environment.
- Speak slowly, clearly; do not shout.
- Explain procedures carefully.
- Face the patient when speaking.
- Use pen and paper for you and patient to assist in communicating.

Non–English-Speaking or Limited Use of the Language

- When patient has no interpreter (friend or family), provide an interpreter.
- Face patient when speaking.
- Speak clearly using short, simple sentences.
- Use visual aids (demonstrations, pictures, gestures).

Visually Impaired

- Announce your presence.
- Offer your arm to guide patient through facility.
- Explain all procedures thoroughly.
- Describe surroundings to the patient.
- If necessary, leave patient alone for only short amounts of time.
- Face the patient when speaking.

Communication Barriers

Disorientation: Loss of memory for time, person, place.
Introjection: Person identifies with attitudes or characteristics of another individual.
Manipulating: Influence, control artfully or deceptively.
Medical terminology: Medical terms and abbreviations should not be used unless explained.
Noise: Interruptions and noise (within room or just outside).
Physical signs/sounds: Facial frown, no eye contact, folded arms/crossed legs, poor voice tone.
Prejudice: Having a negative opinion or bias toward individual.
Stereotyping: Believing all group members (race, religion, etc.) share same attitudes, appearances.

Defense Mechanisms

Denial

- Failure to recognize or acknowledge the existence of anxiety-provoking information.

Displacement

- Redirection of emotional impulses toward a substitute person/object that is less threatening or dangerous.

Inversion

- Patient does opposite of what they want.
- Reverse feelings about someone after being rejected by them.

Projection

- Attributing one's own unacceptable urges or qualities to others.

Rationalization

- Justifying one's actions/feelings with socially acceptable explanations instead of one's true motives/desires.

Reaction Formation

- Thinking/behaving in extreme opposite of unacceptable urges/impulses.

Regression

- Retreat to behavior characteristic of earlier stage of development; i.e., sucking thumb.

Repression

- Complete exclusion from consciousness of anxiety-producing thoughts, feelings, or impulses.
- Basic defense mechanism.

Sublimation

- Displacement form, i.e., sexual urge is rechanneled into productive nonsexual activities.

Suppression

- Deliberate putting aside or forgetting unpleasant past.
- Conscious form of repression.

Telephone Communication

Paralanguage: The way a message is said.

Courtesy

- Etiquette, good manners.
- Respectful treatment of caller.

Diction

- Refers to choice of words, no use of medical jargon/terminology.
- Clarity in pronunciation, no slurring.

Inflection

- A change in pitch.

Pronunciation

- Do this correctly to avoid any misunderstanding.
- Avoid slang and unfamiliar words.

Speed

- Should be a normal rate, not slow or fast.

Tone

- Overall timber and pitch of voice.
- Should have voice sound that is easy to listen to.

Volume

- Keep voice at normal level.
- Always remain calm.

Written Communication

Telephone Message Essentials

- Name of person whom the call is for.
- Date and time of call.
- Name of individual calling.
- Caller's cell phone number, work phone number, home phone number; hours in which to use each number; name and phone number of pharmacy, if needed.
- Detail reason for call.
- Action required (call back, Rx refill, etc.).
- Initials of person taking the message.

Supplies

Paper

- **Bond**
  1. Felt side and wire side and a watermark
  2. 25% or ↑ cotton fiber
- **Weight**
  1. 20–24 lb (↑ number: heavier paper)
  2. 500 sheets per ream

- **Size**
  1. **Standard:** 8.5 × 11 inches (general business correspondence)
  2. **Monarch (executive):** 7.25 × 10.5 inches (office memorandum)
  3. **Baronial:** 5.5 × 8.5 inches (half standard paper sheet)

Envelopes

- **No. 10:** For standard paper
- **6¾:** For baronial paper

Business Letters

Format

Single spaced

Dateline: Keyed on line 15 (no letterhead); 2–3 lines below letterhead.

Inside address: Fourth line below dateline.

Salutation: Second line below inside address; colon follows salutation.

Subject line: Second line below inside address; begin at left margin, indent 5 spaces, or centered.

Body of letter: Second line below salutation or subject line.

Complimentary closing: Second line below last line of body.

Keyed signature: Fourth line below closing.

Reference initials: Left margin, second line below keyed signature; a slash or colon to separate composer and typist; or upper-case composer, lower-case typist.

Enclosure notation: Directly below initials.

Copy notation: Directly below previously typed line.

Postscripts: Second line below previously typed line.

Continuation Page

- Begin 1 inch (line 7) from top of page.
- Required heading information on first keyed line:
  1. Name of addressee.
  2. Page number.
  3. Date.
- Body of letter begins on 10th line from top or third line below heading.

- Complimentary closings:
  1. For a formal style use "respectfully yours" or "respectfully."
  2. For a general style use "very truly yours" or "truly yours"; or "sincerely" or "sincerely yours."
  3. For an informal style (when using first names) use "regards" or "best wishes."

Style

Full block: All typed lines begin at left margin; most efficient but less attractive on page.

Modified block: Typed lines begin at left margin, but date line and complimentary closing are centered.

Indented modified block: New paragraph lines indented 5 spaces (use tab key).

Simplified: All typed lines begin at left margin; omits salutation and complimentary closing; subject line keyed in capital letters on third line below inside address.

Memoranda (Interoffice)

- Begin 2 inches (line 13) from top of page.
- Heading includes date, to, from, subject.

Heading Example #1

TO	All Staff
FROM	Kristen Corrrell, Office Manager
DATE	April 30, 200x
SUBJECT	Summer Staffing Schedule
	I will soon be planning for office staff coverage this upcoming summer season. If you know your summer vacation plans, please submit them at the next scheduled staff meeting on May 12 at 8:30 a.m.

Heading Example #2

MEMO TO: Clinical Supervisor, Claire Lorraine
Administrative Supervisor, JoAnn Carlson

FROM: Jeffrey Daigle, Office Manager

DATE: March 7, 200x

SUBJECT: Office Inventory

The new practice when receiving supplies (office and clinical) from vendors will be as follows:

1. Each box must be clearly marked with the date of receipt.
2. Each box must be numbered (1, 2, 3, etc.)
3. Begin using the highest numbered box. The last box opened will be #1.
4. Orders need not be made until the last box is opened for use.

Envelope (#10)
Spacing, lettering, capitalization, punctuation, notations

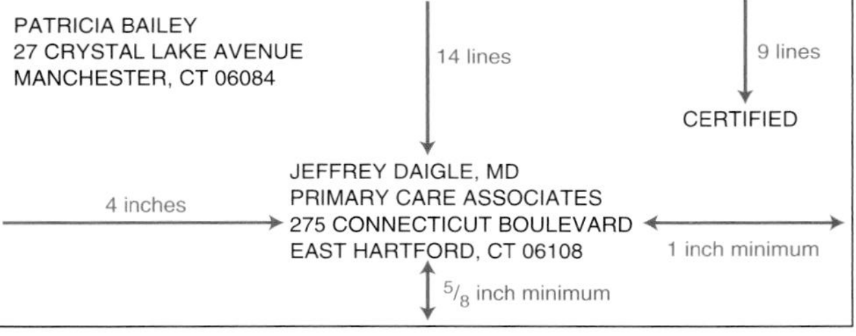

PATRICIA BAILEY
27 CRYSTAL LAKE AVENUE
MANCHESTER, CT 06084
14 lines
9 lines
CERTIFIED
JEFFREY DAIGLE, MD
PRIMARY CARE ASSOCIATES
275 CONNECTICUT BOULEVARD
EAST HARTFORD, CT 06108
4 inches
1 inch minimum
5/8 inch minimum

Envelope (#6 $^3/_4$)
Spacing, lettering, capitalization, punctuation, notations

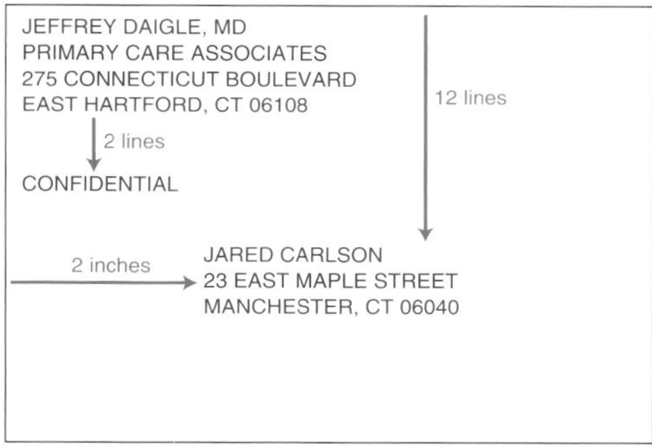

Your Notes

Proofreading Marks

Mark	Meaning	Mark	Meaning
?	is this correct?	⎵	move down
/	delete or change	⎴	move up
^	insert a character	⁐	close up space
≡	set in capital letter(s)	sp	spell out
[	move to the left	⊙	insert period
]	move to the right	¶	new paragraph
#	insert a space	\ or ℘	delete
/ or lc	use lowercase	^,	insert comma

E-mail

- If patient-related, remains confidential, hard copy placed in patient chart.
- To patients: reminder of scheduled appointments for next day.
- Similar to memoranda, often used in place of interoffice memoranda (use the office format).
- No letterhead, inside address, or dateline needed.
- Remaining letter parts used with proper grammar and punctuation.
- Be sure to proofread.

Instant Messages

- Real-time communication.
- To communicate with one another within the office.
- For risk management reasons, this should be checked frequently throughout office hours if:
  1. Setup includes professional contacts outside of office.
  2. Setup includes accessibility to patients (patients must give consent before using e-mail to communicate).

Faxes

- **Cover sheet**: Required, briefly states confidential content, specifically to whom it is directed, number of pages, name and fax number of sender.
- Proper grammar and punctuation.
- Use only when necessary; higher risk of violating patient confidentiality.

Your Notes

Think you got all that?

Test yourself using your enclosed CD-ROM!

Notes

Notes

Notes